MRCP 2:

Neu  for P⸗⸗⸗S

Dr JB Peiris
MD, FRCP (Lond), FRCP (Edin), FRCP (Glas), Hon. FRACP
Consultant Neurologist
(Honorary Foreign Fellow of Association of British Neurologists)

Dr Natasha Peiris
BM (Southampton UK), BSc (Penn., USA)
Registrar in Medicine

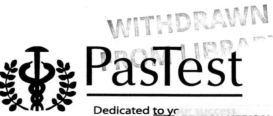

PasTest

Dedicated to your success

© 2002 PASTEST LTD
Egerton Court
Parkgate Estate
Knutsford
Cheshire
WA16 8DX

Telephone: 01565 752000

First published 2002
Reprinted 2002, 2004

ISBN 1 901198 74 X
ISBN 978 19011198 744

A catalogue record for this book is available from the British Library.
The information contained within this book was obtained by the author from reliable sources. However, while every effort has been made to ensure its accuracy, no responsibility for loss, damage or injury occasioned to any person acting or refraining from action as a result of information contained herein can be accepted by the publishers or author.

Every effort has been made to contact holders of copyright to obtain permission to reproduce copyright material. However, if any have been inadvertently overlooked, the publisher will be pleased to make the necessary arrangements at the first opportunity.

PasTest Revision Books and Intensive Courses
PasTest has been established in the field of postgraduate medical education since 1972, providing revision books and intensive study courses for doctors preparing for their professional examinations. Books and courses are available for the following specialities:
MRCP Part 1 and Part 2, MRCPCH Part 1 and Part 2, MRCOG, DRCOG, MRCGP, MRCPsych, DCH, FRCA, MRCS and PLAB.

For further details contact:

PasTest Ltd, Freepost, Knutsford, Cheshire, WA16 7BR
Tel: 01565 752000   **Fax: 01565 650264**
Email: enquiries@pastest.co.uk   Web site: www.pastest.co.uk

Typeset by Saxon Graphics Ltd, Derby
Printed and bound by CPI Antony Rowe, Eastbourne
Cover illustration: Fig 52: UL Dermatomes

Every effort has been made to contact holders of copyright to obtain permission to reproduce copyright material. However, if any have been inadvertently overlooked, the publisher will be pleased to make the necessary arrangements at the first opportunity.

CONTENTS

GLOSSARY

APB	Abductor Pollicis Brevis
ADL	Activities of Daily Living
ADM	Abductor Digiti Minimi
AHC	Anterior Horn Cell
AIDP	Acute Inflammatory Demyelinating Polyradiculopathy
AJ	Ankle Jerk
APB	Abductor Pollicis Brevis
AR	Autosomal Recessive
BJ	Biceps Jerk
CF	Counting Fingers
CNS	Central Nervous System
CPK	Creatine Phosphokinase
CT	Computerised Tomography
CSF	Cerebrospinal Fluid
CTS	Carpal Tunnel Syndrome
DIP	Distal Interphalangeal Joint
DSMA	Distal Spinal Muscular Atrophy
EMG	Electromyogram
ESR	Erythrocyte Sedimentation Rate
FM	Finger Movements
HAM	HTLV1 Associated Myelopathy
IM	Intramuscular
KJ	Knee Jerk
LMN	Lower Motor Neurone
LPS	Levator Palpebrae Superioris
MCP	Metacarpo-Phalangeal Joint
MLB	Medial Longitudinal Bundle
MND	Motor Neurone Disease
MRI	Magnetic Resonance Imaging
MS	Multiple Sclerosis
NPL	No Perception of Light
PACES	Practical Assessment of Clinical Examination Skills
PIP	Proximal Interphalangeal Joint

PL	Perception of Light
RIND	Reversible Ischaemic Neurological Deficit
RTA	Road Traffic Accidents
SACD	Subacute Combined Degeneration of Cord
SAH	Subarachnoid Haemorrhage
SDH	Subdural Haematoma
SJ	Supinator Jerk
SMA	Spinal Muscular Atrophy
SOF	Superior Orbital Fissure
SMON	Subacute Myelo-Optico-Neuropathy
SSPE	Subacute Sclerosing Panencephalitis
SOL	Space-Occupying Lesion
TJ	Triceps Jerk
UMN	Upper Motor Neurone

INTRODUCTION

From June 2001, PACES (Practical Assessment of Clinical Examination Skills) replaced the clinical and viva parts of the MRCP part 2 examination in all centres in the UK.

This is a major change that requires a substantial variation in the method of preparation for the examination. PACES aims to be a more standardised and objective assessment of a candidate's examination skills and a fairer examination overall.

PACES probably requires less depth of knowledge but sharper clinical examination skills that are usually acquired with years of bedside experience.

The MRCP(UK) Part 2 PACES is the clinical part of the MRCP(UK) Part 2 Examination which is now being taken separately from the MRCP(UK) Part 2 Written Examination.

The MRCP Part 2 Written Examination can now be taken at any time within the seven year MRCP Part 1 Regulation Period after a candidate has passed the MRCP Part 1 Examination.

After a candidate has passed the MRCP Part 2 written examination, and providing they have:

- passed their primary qualification two and a half years or more before
- spent at least 12 months in post(s) involving management of unselected medical emergencies within the last five years,

they may sit the MRCP Part 2 PACES.

On passing PACES candidates are entitled to receive the award of MRCP Diploma.

The PACES examination consists of five clinical stations, each assessed by two independent examiners. Candidates start at any of the stations, then move around the carousel (see Fig 1) at 20 minute intervals until they have completed the cycle.

About this Book

This book provides the PACES pre-examination preparation required for **the central nervous system station and history taking** of a neurological patient. It does not deal with the details or technique of examination that a candidate for the MRCP should have mastered.

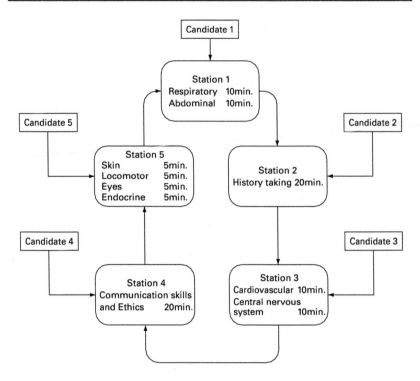

Figure 1: PACES carousel (reproduced with the permission of the Federation of Royal Colleges of Physicians of the UK)

It explains the thinking process involved when the candidate is confronted with a neurological patient. It also provides the background knowledge required with an 'at a glance' pictorial presentation of the possible sites of lesion, which is essential in a neurological diagnosis. The book presumes that the reader can elicit Central Nervous System (CNS) signs confidently.

In the PACES carousel, the candidate may come across a neurological patient either at Station 3 – the Neurological and Cardiovascular station (10 minutes each) or at Station 2 – History taking (20 minutes). See the PACES carousel.

The Neurological Station

A detailed head to toe neurological examination will no longer be required for the 10–minute examination of the neurological patient. Instead, under the watchful eye and the discerning ears of the two independent examiners, the candidate will be expected to obtain the relevant history or physical signs. The candidate will receive written instructions of what is expected of him/her.

However, it must be realised that during the 10 minutes at the neurology station, the candidate must carry out a meaningful examination. They will not usually be interrupted by the examiners on the relevance of the particular physical sign for diagnosis, management and prognosis. This station will examine the clinical facets tested in the long case, short case and spots. As such, there is very little time for 'on the spot' analysis of the presentation and prior preparation becomes essential.

The History Taking Skills Station – 20 minutes

The history taking skills station aims to assess the candidate's ability to gather data from the patient, to assimilate information and then discuss the case. The 20 minutes at this station will enable the examiners to assess aspects originally tested in the long case and viva.

This station would have:
- Written instructions for the case, usually in the form of a letter from the patient's GP, given to the candidate during the five–minute interval before the station
- 15 minutes for the history taking followed by five minutes for discussion (after the candidate has left the station)
- Two examiners present throughout to observe history taking
- A structured mark sheet that is marked independently by the two examiners

General Guidelines and Helpful Hints

The new format of the examination will require the candidate to be quick thinking and more clinically orientated.

It is essential to have a good knowledge of the probable diagnosis and differential diagnosis of the neurological conditions to be found at the neurological and history taking stations.

This book sets out such background knowledge step-by-step. It also teaches the analytical process needed to elicit physical signs in a way that will enable one possibility to be differentiated from another. When eliciting each physical sign, the candidate should aim to either confirm or exclude a particular site of lesion or disorder.

This book is divided into neurology and history taking stations to help candidates follow the step-by-step diagnosis.

There are three stages of diagnosis.

Three Stages of Diagnosis

1   **Site**: Where is the lesion?
2   **Nature**: What is the lesion?
3   **Cause**: How or why was the lesion caused?

The nature of the symptoms and elicited signs are useful in determining the site, while the temporal profile (duration, onset and progress) is helpful in determining the nature.

The previous history, social and family history, investigations, epidemiology, etc may indicate the possible cause/s.

If the three stage diagnosis is kept in mind, it will not be difficult to have a reasonable concept of the diagnosis or at least the possibilities (differential diagnosis) at the end of history taking. In this book, for certain presentations the analysis may be over-simplified so that the clinical problem can be easily understood.

The candidate is strongly advised to read the section on localised weakness which follows and the differential qualities of upper and lower motor neurone lesions at different sites (see pages 7–23) before going on to the individual presentations.

Acknowledgements

Some of the illustrations are modified from Aids to the Examination of the Peripheral Nervous System, 4th edition, The Guarantors of Brain 2000, W B Saunders, London.

MOTOR DISTURBANCES IN LIMBS

LOCALISED WEAKNESS

THE DIFFERENCE BETWEEN LOWER MOTOR NEURONE (LMN) LESIONS AND UPPER MOTOR NEURONE (UMN) LESIONS

Weakness of:

- a limb/s
- part of a limb
- individual muscle/s supplied by spinal or cranial nerves

is the most common clinical neurological presentation for clinical examinations.

Irrespective of the nature of the symptom, the first step in the examination is to determine whether it is a lower motor neurone (LMN) or upper motor neurone (UMN) lesion.

The exact location of the lesion in the efferent pathway of the reflex arc or the site of the pathology in the pyramidal pathway is then determined.

Examination of the motor system alone is often sufficient to determine whether it is a LMN or UMN lesion or a combination of both.

Functional or non-organic disorders can mimic either or a combination of both, and the candidate may need to have a lot of experience to make a diagnosis of a functional disorder with confidence.

Lesions at the level of muscle and neuro-muscular junction have features similar to LMN lesions though they cannot strictly be classified as LMN.

The Difference between LMN Lesions and UMN Lesions

	LMN TYPE	UMN TYPE
Wasting	+	−
Tone	hypotonic	hypertonic
Power	proportionate reduction*	disproportionate reduction**
Reflexes	+/−	++
Abdominals	+	−
Plantars	flexor/absent	extensor

*Reduction in muscle power (weakness elicited) is proportionate to disability.
** Weakness elicited is less than disability.
(This explanatory note is important – see also page 10.)

Having decided whether it is a LMN or UMN lesion or a combination of both, it is essential to determine the level of lesion.

Parameters to Determine Level of LMN Lesion

- **Motor level**: Wasting and weakness
- **Sensory Level**: Root or spinal
- **Reflex Level**: Level of impaired reflex or most cephalad brisk reflex

The five sites of lesion, which produce a LMN type of clinical picture (see Fig 2) are:

- Muscle
- Neuro-muscular junction
- Mixed spinal nerve
- Ventral root
- Anterior horn cell – motor neurone

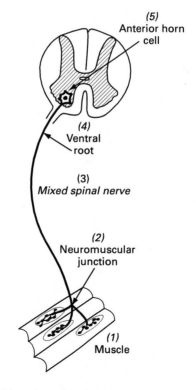

Figure 2: Sites for flaccid weakness/wasting

Levels of LMN Type Clinical Picture

SITE	CLINICAL ENTITY
1 Muscle	Myopathy
2 Neuromuscular	Myasthenia
Junction	Gravis
3 Nerve	Neuropathy
4 Nerve root	Radiculopathy
5 Motor neurone	Diseases of motor neurone
	(Polio, MND, SMA – Spinal Muscular Atrophy)

Motor Level – Determination by Distribution of Wasting

Wasting is absent in UMN lesions except in so-called 'parietal wasting' (in cerebral palsy) and due to disuse atrophy. Wasting is present in chronic or subacute LMN or muscle disorders. The distribution of wasting depends on the site of pathology.

Site of lesion	Distribution of wasting	Condition
Muscle	Proximal and symmetrical	Myopathy
Nerve	Localised or distal and symmetrical	Neuropathy
Nerve root	Dermatomal	Radiculopathy
Plexus	Whole limb, proximal or distal part of a limb	Brachial or lumbo-sacral plexopathy
Anterior horn cell	Dermatomal	Disease of motor neurone

Lesions at the level of neuro-muscular junction (myasthenia) may rarely produce symmetrical and proximal wasting late in the disease, at which time myasthenic features can be absent (myasthenic myopathy).

Motor Level – Fasciculation

This is absent in UMN lesions. It occurs in the progressive disease of motor neurone as in motor neurone disease (MND), spinal muscular atrophy (SMA) and syringomyelia. The fasciculation is often limited to the 'actively wasting' muscles.

Motor Level – Tone

Tone is hypotonic or flaccid in LMN and hypertonic or spastic in UMN lesions. It is shown by passive movements at the knee, ankle, elbow and wrist. 'Clasp knife' spasticity may be demonstrated in the legs by lifting a leg with the hand behind the lower thigh.

Motor Level – Power

The degree of weakness depends on the severity of the condition. In LMN lesions the functional disability is **proportionate** to the weakness elicited on examination. In UMN lesion the weakness shown by examining individual muscles is **disproportionate** to the disability.

Spasticity adds a further element of disability to the demonstrable weakness. For example, a patient with a severe spastic paraparesis due to spinal cord compression who is unable to walk may have near normal muscle power on the testing of individual lower limb muscles.

On the other hand, a patient with a flaccid foot drop due to a common peroneal palsy will have difficulty in dorsi-flexing the feet even against gravity. It is useful to note that LMN lesions affect the power of individual muscles (e.g. weakness of dorsiflexors in foot drop) but UMN lesions produce weakness of a movement (e.g. weakness of arm and leg in hemiplegia).

Reflex Level

- **LMN**: Reflex at the level of the lesion is diminished or absent, depending on the reflex arc affected
- **UMN**: Reflexes below level of lesion are brisk

Reflex	Root/level	Nerve of supply
Biceps (BJ)	C5, C6	Musculo-cutaneous
Supinator (SJ)	C5, C6	Radial
Triceps (TJ)	C6, C7, C8	Radial
Knee (KJ)	L2, L3, L4	Femoral
Ankle (AJ)	S1	Tibial
Plantar	S1	Tibial
Abdominal	T7–T12	Intercostal
Cremasteric	L2	Obturator

Note: The L5 nerve root is not involved in any reflex.

Sensory 'Level'

While UMN lesions may show a sensory level, LMN lesions show localised impairment or loss of sensation – distal, root or nerve in distribution. Lesions at muscle, NMJ, AHC levels do not have sensory signs.

Sensory Level – UMN Lesions

For lesions in the cervical and thoracic cord, look carefully for a level in the upper limbs, chest or abdomen.

SENSORY LEVEL	SITE OF LEVEL
C5 – T1	Upper limb/s
T2 – T7	Chest (Rib cage, anterior or posterior)
T2	Angle of Louis
T4	Male nipple level
T7	Xiphisternum
T7 – T12	Front of abdomen
L1	Groin
S2,3	Genitalia

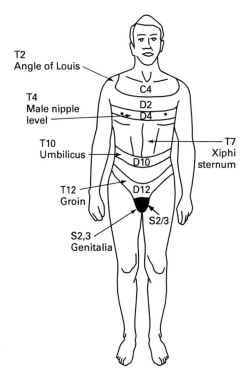

Figure 3: Sensory levels

Sensory Level (Loss) in LMN Lesions

- **Glove and stocking**: Peripheral neuropathies
- **Dermatomal**: In nerve root lesions
- **Localised**: To sensory distribution of affected nerve

Special Sensory Loss

- **Intramedullary**: 'Dissociate sensory loss'. Pain and temperature is affected while touch is preserved.
- **Extra-medullary and extra dural**: There is a sensory loss over the saddle area in the back.

LOWER MOTOR NEURONE (LMN) TYPE LESIONS

Though all LMN lesions have features in common described on page 7 there are additional features specific to the level or site of lesion, e.g. nerve, nerve root, plexus or neurone. Irrespective of the symptom or cause shown, there are features common to a particular site of LMN lesion.

Feature of Lesions at Level of Muscle – Myopathy

Wasting and weakness are proximal and symmetrical involving the shoulder girdle and hip girdle. Reflexes may be preserved till late, e.g. ankle jerk. The weakness shown on examination will be proportionate to the disability.

In the **inherited non-inflammatory myopathies**, the onset is insidious and the wasting and weakness is slowly progressive.

In the **inflammatory myopathies** the proximal muscles may show the classical signs of inflammation – red, hot, painful, swelling with loss of function – rubor, calor, dolor, tumor and functio laesa.

Muscle enzymes (CPK, Aldolase) are usually elevated. EMG is characteristic showing low voltage and a poor recruitment pattern. Metabolic and other causes need to be looked for in the acquired varieties.

Features of Lesions at Level of Neuromuscular Junction — Myasthenia Gravis

The hallmark of myasthenia is fatigability of the affected muscle/s. Commonly affected muscles are:

- **Ocular:** Asymmetrical ptosis and diplopia with or without ocular paresis

- **Bulbar:** Dysarthria, dysphagia, nasal voice and regurgitation
- **Limb/s:** Commonly proximal but could be distal or global
- **General:** Ocular, bulbar and limb. Wasting of proximal muscles may be seen after many years (myasthenic myopathy) when features of myasthenia may be absent.

Nerve – Neuropathy

Clinically this may affect a single nerve (mono-neuropathy), multiple nerves (mononeuritis multiplex), many nerves diffusely (polyneuropathy) or distal nerves (peripheral neuropathy). The affection may be mainly motor, sensory or a combination of the two – sensory-motor neuropathy.

- **Motor:** May not affect all muscles supplied
- **Sensory:** Usually numbness rather than pain and the symptom may not be well sited to the sensory distribution of nerve, e.g. it may involve the whole hand in the carpal tunnel syndrome.
- **Reflex:** Impaired or absent

Nerve Root – Radiculopathy

Clinically the nerve root means the first part of the mixed spinal nerve and dorsal and ventral nerve roots do not need to be considered separately. The nerve root is often affected by disc prolapse. Clinically, commonly affected nerve roots are:

- **Upper limbs:** C5, C6, T1, less commonly C7, C8
- **Lower limbs:** L5,S1, less commonly L4, and S2–S4.

Diffuse affection of nerve roots occurs in the polyradiculopathy of the Guillain Barré type.

Motor Radiculopathy

Weakness and wasting corresponds to the supply of the particular nerve root.

- **C5, C6:** Shoulder girdle
- **C7, C8:** Flexors of wrist and fingers
- **T1:** Intrinsic hand muscles
- **L5:** Dorsiflexion of foot and toes
- **S1:** Plantar flexion and eversion

Lumbo-sacral nerve roots may be affected in the spinal canal or pelvis (see Fig 5).

Sensory Radiculopathy

Unlike neuropathy, radiculopathy is often present with pain. The radiation of pain is fairly classical. It can be detected more in the lower limbs, but less so in the upper ones.

- **L5** – pain radiates from lower back → buttocks → outer thigh → outer calf → dorsum of foot → big toe
- **S1–** lower back → buttocks → back of thigh → back of calf → heel → little toe
- **C5, C6** – side of neck → outer upper arm → outer forearm → thumb, index finger
- **C8, T1** – side of neck → arm → inner forearm → little and ring finger

When there are bilateral root pains at the same level in the chest or abdomen, a tightening 'band-like' sensation is produced at that level, called 'girdle pains'. Girdle pains usually indicate a compressive lesion at that level. Bilateral sciatica involving the same bilateral roots has the same significance and is often produced by a large central disc prolapse.

Plexus Lesions
- **Brachial:** C5 – T1
- **Lumbo-sacral:** L1–S5

These are usually unilateral and incomplete. Pain may be severe. The motor and sensory features depend on the nerve root/s affected.

Neuronal Lesions
The anterior horn cell (AHC) or cranial nerve nuclei are affected.

- **Sensory:** Nil
- **Motor:** Same as for nerve root or cranial nerve
- **Reflexes:** Diminished or absent at the level

UPPER MOTOR NEURONE TYPE LESIONS

Though all UMN lesions have certain features in common described on page 7 there are other specific features which enable the site of lesion in the pyramidal or cortico–spinal pathway to be found accurately.

Clinically lesions are considered at the following levels (Fig 4).

Sites of UMN Lesions

Spinal cord:

- Lumbar: Opposite L1 vertebra
- Thoracic: T1 –T12
- Cervical: C1– C7
- Foramen magnum

Brain stem:

- Medulla
- Pons
- Mid brain

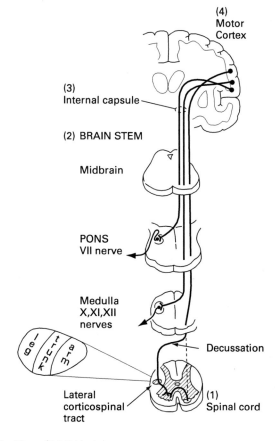

Figure 4: Sites of UMN lesions

Internal capsule site

Cortex site

In the examination of UMN lesions it is important to look at all long tracts.

Long tracts

- **Pyramidal:** Spastic weakness and hyper-reflexia on the side of the weakness with extensor plantars
- **Spinothalamic:** Loss of pain and temperature below the lesion on the opposite side
- **Posterior column:** Loss of position and vibration sense on the same side

The parameters assessed to determine the level of a UMN lesion are the same as those to assess a LMN lesion, namely motor, sensory and reflex levels.

Parameters to Assess UMN Lesions

- Motor level
- Sensory level
- Reflex level

UMN Lesions in Spinal Cord

Lumbar Level

As the spinal cord ends at the lower border of L1 vertebra, lesions below L1 will not produce UMN signs. Opposite the L1 vertebra, L1 – S5 nerve roots of both sides surround the bottom of the spinal cord. Lesions at L1 produce a conus medullaris or 'high cauda equina ' lesion (see Fig 5).

At this level both the spinal cord and nerve roots may be affected. Any or all of the lumbo-sacral nerve roots may be damaged unilaterally or bilaterally, particularly with trauma. There may also be UMN signs in the form of brisk ankle jerk (AJ) and extensor plantars, but reflexes may be impaired depending on the nerve roots involved.

Motor: Spastic paraparesis (after initial flaccid phase in trauma). Wasting and LMN weakness may be present depending on the roots affected.

Reflexes: AJ may be brisk with extensor plantar. Sphincteric reflexes may be absent.

Sensory: There is variable sensory loss in the legs and sacral area. Position sense may be affected depending on the site of the lesion.

(lateral view)

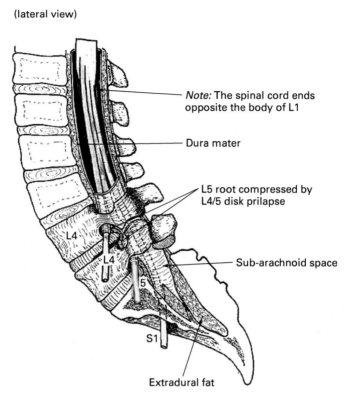

Figure 5: Cauda equina

Thoracic Level

T1 – T12: This is a common site of lesion in spastic paraplegia due to compressive lesions.

Motor: Arms are unaffected. There are features of a spastic paraparesis in the legs – spastic weakness is disproportionate to the evident disability. The power of individual muscles may be almost normal though there is a significant difficulty in walking.

Beevor's sign: A lesion at T10 spinal level causes the umbilicus to be drawn upwards when the head is flexed.

Reflexes: There is a brisk knee jerk (KJ), AJ with extensor plantars. The abdominals may help to localise the lesion between T7 and T12.

Sensory level: In spastic paraparesis, a sensory level is often detectable on the chest or abdomen due to a thoracic cord lesion (see Fig 3). There is a sacral

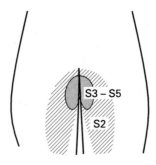

Figure 6: Saddle sensory loss

sensory loss in the 'saddle area' (see Fig 6) in extradural lesions. Posterior column sensation may be affected depending on the site of the lesion.

Sensory Landmarks

- **Angle of Louis:** T2
- **Male nipple:** T4
- **Xiphisternum:**T7

- **Umbilicus:** T10
- **Inguinal ligament:** T12

As the spinal cord is shorter than the vertebral column, (Fig 7), the spinal level as determined by the neurological examination should be co-related to the vertebral level. This can be detected by tenderness, kyphosis and imaging.

Spinal and Vertebral Levels Compared

VERTEBRAL LEVEL	SPINAL LEVEL
C7	C8 (add 1)
T5	T7 (add 2)
T9	T12 (add 3)
T10	L1, L2
T11 ·	L3, L4
T12–L1	L5–S5

Cervical Level

Motor: In addition to the UMN signs in the legs similar to the thoracic level lesion, there may be wasting or weakness of the neck or upper limb muscles on one or both sides. Upper level of dermatomal weakness denotes the level of lesion.

Sensory: Determine a level in the neck or upper limb/s at C2 – T1 level. There is a sacral sensory loss in extradural lesions (see Fig 6). Posterior columns may be affected.

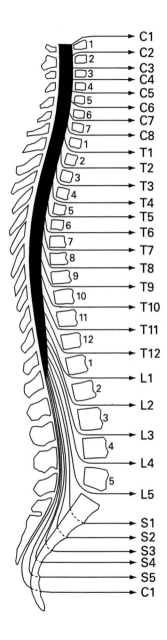

Figure 7: Spinal cord in relation to vertebral column

Reflexes: The highest level of impaired or absent reflex indicates a reflex level of lesion, e.g. impaired or absent BJ and SJ with brisk TJ occurs in C5, C6 lesions. Reflexes below this level will be exaggerated. It is important to look specifically for inverted SJ, i.e. finger flexion without brachio-radialis contraction on eliciting SJ.

Foramen Magnum Level

Motor: All four limbs are weak. They may be asymmetrical and incomplete.

Sensory: This may be detectable in the occiput or neck – C2, C3, C4. (Note – there is no C1 sensory dermatome.) Posterior columns may be affected depending on the location of the lesion.

Reflexes: All UL and LL reflexes are brisk. Additional signs indicative of a cranio-spinal lesion may be mirror movements and downbeat nystagmus on horizontal gaze.

UMN Lesions at Brain Stem Level

As for cervical and cranio-spinal lesions, there will be a spastic quadriparesis with or without other long tract signs. Also, depending on the site of the lesion, cranial nerve nuclei may be affected as indicated.

Cranial Nerve Nuclei in Brain Stem

- **Medulla:** IX–XII
- **Pons:** V–VIII
- **Mid Brain:** III, IV

There would be corresponding symptoms and appropriate motor, sensory and reflex signs would be elicited.

A crossed hemiplegia is of immense localising significance. Crossed hemiplegia is a LMN cranial nerve palsy of one side with a contra-lateral hemiparesis. It indicates where the lesion is located – at the site and side of the cranial nerve involved.

For example, R. III palsy with L. hemiparesis (Weber's syndrome) indicates a lesion of the R. mid brain (see Fig 11 on page 22).

A lesion of the R. pons produces a L. hemiparesis and conjugate weakness to the same (right) side, i.e. the head and eyes will deviate to the left or paralysed side. (Remember – as with pontine lesions – head and eyes are to the paralysed side.)

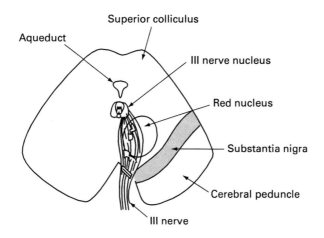

Figure 8: Mid brain

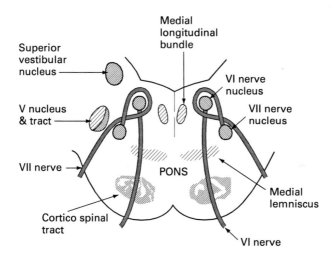

Figure 9: Pons

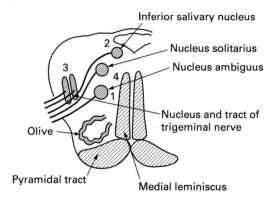

Figure 10: Medulla

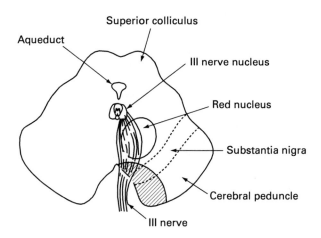

Figure 11: Weber's syndrome

Internal Capsular Lesions

These are usually unilateral, unless there have been two separate lesions at different times. They produce a UMN face-arm-leg paresis of the opposite side. They are usually vascular with intact speech (may be slurred) and are rarely accompanied by hemi-anaesthesia and hemianopia (see Fig 12).

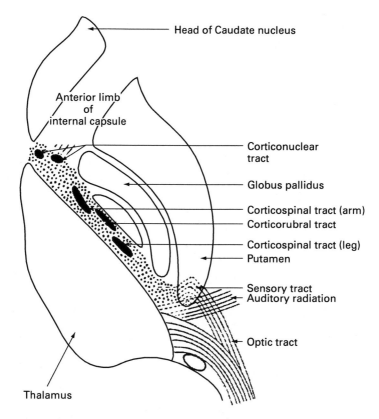

Figure 12: Internal capsule

Cortical Lesions

Cortical lesions involving paracentral motor cortex will produce a contralateral spastic hemiparesis. A para-sagittal lesion will produce a spastic paraparesis. There may be an associated cortical sensory loss (see pages 164–165).

Cortical lesions not producing any weakness are dealt with separately later, under disorders of vision and disorders of speech.

PARAPLEGIA AND PARAPARESIS

NEUROLOGY STATION

The general comments under localised weakness (see pages 7–23) should be read along with this section.

Features and causes depend on whether it is a flaccid (LMN) or a spastic (UMN) paraplegia. Acute UMN lesions (trauma, myelitis) are initially flaccid and may take days or weeks to develop UMN signs. So signs also depend on the duration of paraparesis.

	FLACCID	SPASTIC
Wasting	+	0
Tone	hypotonic	hypertonic
Power	proportionate	disproportionate
	to disability	to disability
KJ	diminished	++
AJ	or absent	++
Abdominals	+ +	absent
Cremasteric	+ +	absent
Plantars	flexor/absent	extensor
Sensation	normal, saddle	sensory level +/-
	or peripheral	chest or abdomen

To complete the 'list' of causes, first consider them according to clinical importance and frequency of occurrence, and then by site of the lesion.

Spinal Cord Compression

Read the section on UMN lesions at the spinal cord level – thoracic and lumbar 1 (pages 16–20). Cord compression can happen at any age though pathology differs with age.

Spinal cord compression may be:

1   Intra-medullary

2 Extra-medullary
- intradural
- extradural

Intramedullary: Commonly glioma, ependymoma

Extradural: Bone lesions – myeloma, secondaries

Intradural extramedullary: With or without extradural extension or totally extradural: Meningioma, neurofibroma, lymphomas

There are six clinical presentations:

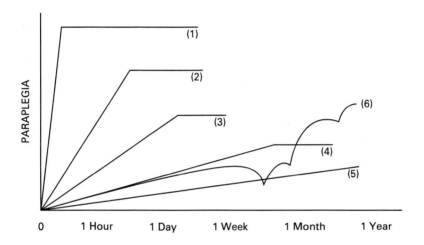

	Nature	Timescale	Condition/s
1	Ultra acute	Instant or minutes	Vertebral collapse, vascular
2	Acute	Within 24 hours	Polio, toxic, metabolic
3	Subacute	1–3 days	Epidural abscess
4	Progresses to plateau and improves	1–4 weeks for maximal deficit	Guillain Barré syndrome Transverse myelitis
5	'Chronic' progressive	Months or years	Classical cord compression myopathy, degenerative disorders, neuropathies, some neuronal (MND)
6	Remittent or stepwise	Variable	Demyelination (MS)

Figure 13: Temporal profile of paraplegia

1 Classical: Insidious onset, progressive (usually months) spastic, hyper-reflexic paraparesis, often with a sensory level and bladder involvement.

2 Ultra acute: Usually traumatic or neoplastic, associated with destructive collapse of vertebra. Onset may be ultra acute (seconds or minutes). The paraplegia is often dense, initially flaccid with retention and the sensory level. Later spastic paraplegia with hyper-reflexia is similar to the 'classical variety'.

3 Subacute: It is clinically very important to recognise at an early stage a rapidly progressive paraparesis over a few hours. This is because a rapidly developing epidural abscess will need urgent decompression. The signs will be those of a spastic paraparesis.

4 Progressive with arrest and improvement: Maximal onset occurs in a few days or weeks, and usually does not exceed a month. After a plateau phase there is improvement.

5 Step-by-step or 'add-on' weakness: Paraparesis may have progressed in a step-by-step or 'add-on' manner or be slowly progressive. It is seen classically in multiple sclerosis.

Multiple Sclerosis

Look for cerebellar and posterior column signs in particular. There may be a history of visual impairment due to optic or retro-bulbar neuritis or dissemination of neurological symptoms in time and space, i.e. affection of other parts of the CNS at different times.

Signs will be those of a spastic paraparesis with added visual, sensory and cerebellar signs.

Transverse Myelitis

There is a subacute onset, from a few days to a few weeks. There is often an asymmetrical paraparesis, with sensory level and bladder involvement. Initially it may be flaccid and areflexic, later spastic and hyper-reflexic. Usually there is a slow recovery commencing a week or two after the maximal deficit, though recovery may be incomplete.

Cauda Equina Lesion

There is an insidious, progressive, below knee wasting and weakness, with or without bladder involvement and saddle sensory loss. It may be asymmetrical. If the lesion is high (between T10 and L2) KJ are brisk. Ankle jerks are often absent. Onset and progress will depend on the cause of the lesion.

Non-Compressive Myelopathy

Presentation is very similar to spinal cord compression with an insidious, progressive, spastic paraparesis with or without a sensory level. Investigations reveal no cord compression.

Consider the following:

- SACD: Subacute combined degeneration of cord
- Motor neurone disease
- SMA (spinal muscular atrophy): UMN signs minimal or absent
- HAM: HTLV1 associated myelopathy
- SMON (subacute myelo-optico-neuropathy)
- Tropical spastic paraplegia
- HIV/AIDS myelopathy.

Polyneuropathy

This may be acute (toxic exposure), subacute or chronic (metabolic).
There is a peripheral, symmetrical, sensory-motor, flaccid weakness with absent AJ and KJ (or impaired). Sensory loss is distal with an impaired position and vibration sense. Distal wasting may occur later. Sphincters are not affected. Family history is important in hereditary sensory motor neuropathies.

Myopathy

This often occurs in a child or young adult. There is an insidious, progressive, proximal and symmetrical, flaccid weakness with a waddling gait and Gower's climbing up sign. Wasting may be evident. Reflexes can be elicited until late in the disease. Sensation and sphincters are normal. Tenderness arises in polymyositis.

Anterior Spinal Artery Thrombosis

This consists of acute paraplegia in an adult with dissociated sensory level, i.e. touch is unaffected and position sense is preserved, with a level for pain and temperature. Initially weakness is flaccid, later it becomes spastic.

Parasagittal Tumour

This is similar to a cord compression at thoracic level but no sensory level is evident on the chest or abdomen. The bladder may be affected. It may be difficult to find loss of cortical sense in the legs. Joint position sense and vibration sense may be affected.

Parasagittal Tumour vs Thoracic Cord Compression

Although sites are wide apart and investigations required are totally different, it is not always easy to differentiate between a parasagittal tumour and thoracic cord compression. This is because there are many features in common.

PARASAGITTAL TUMOUR	THORACIC CORD COMPRESSION
	Spastic paraparesis
	Insidious, progressive
	Upper limbs spared
	Bladder may be involved
	Position sense may be affected
Intracranial symptoms +/–	Spinal symptoms +/-
Headache, focal fits	Girdle pains
Cortical sensory loss in legs	Sensory level with or without sacral sensory loss

Paraplegia by Site of Lesion

SITE	CONDITION
Muscle	Myopathy
NMJ	Myasthenia
Nerve	Polyneuropathy
Nerve root	Polyradiculopathy of Guillain Barré type
Anterior horn cell	Poliomyelitis
Spinal cord	Inflammation, vascular, tumours
Cortex	Parasagittal lesions – tumour, vascular

Note: Myasthenia is rarely present as paraplegia though in theory it is possible. AIDP (acute inflammatory demyelinating polyradiculopathy) of the Guillain Barré type usually produces a quadriparesis and rarely causes paraplegia. Brain stem lesions produce a quadriparesis or crossed hemiplegia while internal capsular lesions produce a hemiparesis or hemiplegia.

HISTORY TAKING STATION

A good history of the patient is invaluable in determining the nature and cause of the paraplegia. Physical signs help to localise the site of the lesion. At the end of the history the candidate must be able to draw a temporal profile of the paraplegia (see Fig 13 on page 25). It is also important to take a holistic approach to the patient and ask them questions on activities of daily living (ADL).

Specific points to note in the history include the following.

Time Frame

Onset

How long did it take for the maximal deficit to occur – instantaneous, a few hours, days, weeks or months?

Progress

From the onset to present day, is it improving, static or getting worse?

Temporal Profile

From the onset and progress it should be possible to draw a graph of the temporal profile of the paraplegia with paraplegia on the 'y' axis and time on the 'x' axis. This may fit in with the presentations shown in Fig 13 on page 25.

Duration

The time that has lapsed from the start of the paraplegia until the time of examination is not of much importance for diagnosis, once the onset, progress and temporal profile have been determined. However, this is the answer to the usual question of 'How long have you had this ailment?'

Spatial Localisation

Motor

Is the weakness global, proximal or distal? It may be possible to determine the nature of the gait by questioning the patient (without examining, which is not allowed at the history taking station). Is there any difficulty in walking? If so, what is the difficulty?

- **Weak and floppy:** Flaccid weakness
- **High stepping:** Distal weakness
- **Stamping with a need to look down while walking:** Sensory loss
- **Difficulty in getting up and climbing:** Proximal weakness
- **Unsteady:** Cerebellar component (uncommon in true paraplegia)
- **Stiff:** Wading through mud or water – spastic
- **Upper limbs and bulbar muscles:** Are they affected?

Sensory

Ask specifically for:

- Pain in spine
- Girdle pain

- Radicular pain – radiating pain down leg
- Sensory impairment – commonly distal
- Sensory level – a 'cut-off level' below which the patient does not feel pain or other sensation.

Sphincter disturbances

An assessment of the bladder, bowel and sexual functions needs to be carried out during the history. An accurate evaluation of the disturbance in the physiology of micturition can be achieved by asking the patient the following questions. This helps in determining whether the lesion is in the afferent pathway, the inhibitory or facilitatory pathway of micturition.

- Do you get the desire to pass urine? (This is an appreciation of bladder fullness.)
- Can you 'hold your water'?
- Do you need to rush to pass water?
- Have you been incontinent on such an occasion? (Focus on incontinence.)
- Do you have difficulty in starting urination?
- When you urinate does the stream break up or do you have to start again? Do you have a discontinuous stream?
- When you finish, do you still feel that there is more to pass? (This is residual urine.)
- Have you had retention and been catheterised?

Similar questions could be asked on the emptying of the bowel but these become of secondary importance unless faecal incontinence becomes a problem. Usually, how the patient's bladder is functioning is adequate to obtain a reasonable idea of neurological bowel dysfunction.

The patient may not volunteer details about sexual dysfunction but it is necessary to assess:

- Failure of erection
- Failure of sustained erection
- Ejaculatory disturbance – is it premature or delayed?

After focusing on the details of the paraparesis in the complaint along with the history of the patient, do not forget that there may be important clues from:

- Past history
- Family history
- Occupational history
- Social history.

Therapeutic history

At the end of the 15 minutes of history taking, you must be well prepared with the:

- Probable diagnosis with reasons
- Differential diagnosis
- Investigations
- Plan of management
- Résumé to be conveyed to the patient, relatives and GP.

QUADRIPLEGIA AND QUADRIPARESIS

NEUROLOGY STATION

Before starting this chapter read the general comments on localised weakness (see pages 7–23). Quadriparesis can be considered on lines similar to paraplegia, with involvement of all four limbs instead of legs only.

As for paraplegia, features and causes depend on whether it is flaccid (LMN type) or spastic (UMN). Acute UMN lesions (trauma and myelitis at cervical cord level) are initially flaccid and show features of UMN lesions only days or weeks later. So signs depend not only on the level of lesion but also on duration. Paraplegia was considered according to how often the disorder occurred.

For a better and broader understanding of neurological lesions consider quadriparesis according to the site of the lesion, as follows.

LMN Lesions

Muscle level – Myopathies

This often occurs in a child or young adult, mainly affecting the hip and shoulder girdle, usually due to a limb girdle dystrophy. There is an insidious, progressive, proximal and symmetrical, flaccid weakness of the upper and lower limbs with a waddling gait and a Gower's climbing up sign.

The patient has difficulty moving the shoulder while finger movements may not be affected. Wasting may be present in the shoulder, hip and thigh muscles. There may be pseudo-hypertrophy of some muscles – notably the calf and deltoids. Reflexes are detectable till late in the disease. Sensation and sphincters are normal. Tenderness may be present in polymyositis.

Neuromuscular junction – Myasthenia

Myasthenia seldom, if ever, presents itself as quadriplegia but it could be detected as a weakness of all four limbs in the general form. The feature is fatigability with diurnal variation. The ocular and bulbar muscles may be affected.

Nerve level – Polyneuropathy

This may be acute (toxic exposure), subacute or chronic (metabolic). There is a peripheral, symmetrical, sensory-motor, flaccid weakness with absent or impaired jerks in all limbs. Distal sensory loss with impaired position and vibration sense may be seen, particularly in the legs. Distal wasting may be seen later. Sphincters are not affected. Family history is important in hereditary sensory motor neuropathies.

Nerve root level – Polyradiculopathy

This is commonly AIDP (Acute Inflammatory Demyelinating Polyradiculopathy) of the Guillain Barré type, producing a progressive quadriparesis within days or usually a maximum of four weeks. Sensory symptoms precede the weakness and often there is LMN facial paralysis. Ventilatory failure may supervene.

Motor Neurone – Anterior Horn Cell

The conditions needing consideration are:

- Motor neurone disease
- Spinal muscular atrophy
- Syringomyelia
- Poliomyelitis.

Apart from poliomyelitis, other conditions are insidious and progressive. Sensory symptoms and signs are absent in all.

UMN lesions

Cervical Level

The following conditions need to be considered:

- Spinal cord compression – commonly spondylotic
- Trauma
- Myelitis
- Anterior spinal artery thrombosis.

Motor

In addition to the UMN signs in legs there may be wasting or weakness of the neck or upper limb muscles on one or both sides. The upper level of dermatomal weakness is the level of the lesion.

Sensory

Determine a level in the neck or upper limb/s, C2 – T1 level (see Fig 32 on page 83). Sacral sensory loss is present in extradural lesions. Posterior columns may be affected.

Reflexes

The highest level of impaired or absent reflex denotes the reflex level of lesion, e.g. impaired or absent BJ and SJ with brisk TJ indicates a C5, C6 lesion. Reflexes below this level will be exaggerated. It is important to look specifically for inverted SJ – where there is finger flexion without brachio-radialis contraction on eliciting SJ.

Above C5 Level

Motor

There is a spastic weakness of all four limbs.

Sensory

At C2 level it is at the back of the neck. At C3, C4 levels it is at the side of the neck, and angle of the mandible.

Reflexes

All limb reflexes are brisk with extensor plantars, absent abdominal and cremasteric reflexes.

At C5 Level

Motor

Wasting and weakness of deltoid, spinati (supraspinatus and infraspinatus) and biceps.

Sensory

This is at the outer upper arm.

Reflexes

BJ is impaired or absent, SJ is diminished, absent or inverted, TJ is brisk.

At C6 level

Motor

There is a weakness of the brachioradialis.

Sensory

This is at the outer forearm, thumb and index finger.

Reflexes

There is a diminished or absent SJ.

At C7 level

Motor

There is a weakness of long flexors.

Sensory

This is at the middle finger.

Reflex

TJ may be diminished.

C8/T1 Level

Motor

There is a weakness of the interossei, thenar (APB– abductor pollicis brevis), and hypothenar (ADM – Abductor Digiti Minimi) muscles. There may be a claw hand.

Sensory

This affects the ulnar aspect of the ring finger, little finger and inner aspect of the forearm to the elbow.

Reflex

TJ may be diminished.

Summary of C5, C6, C7, C8 T1 Lesions

	MUSCLE	SENSORY	REFLEX
C5	Deltoid, spinati, biceps	Outer upper arm	BJ, SJ diminished
C6	Biceps, brachioradialis	Thumb, index	Diminished BJ, SJ
C7	Long flexors	Middle finger	Diminished TJ
C8/T1	Interossei, APB, ADM	Ulnar 1 1/2 fingers	Diminished TJ inner forearm

Foramen Magnum Level

Motor

There is a weakness of all four limbs. It may be asymmetrical and incomplete.

Sensory

This may be detectable in the occiput or neck – C2, C3, C4. (There is no C1 sensory dermatome.) Posterior columns may be affected depending on the extent of the lesion.

Reflexes

All UL and LL reflexes are brisk. Additional signs indicating a cranio-spinal lesion may be mirror movements and downbeat nystagmus on a horizontal gaze.

Brain Stem Level

As for cervical and cranio-spinal lesions, there will be a spastic quadriparesis with or without other long tract signs. Also, depending on the site of the lesion, the cranial nerve nuclei may be affected as indicated here:

Cranial Nerve Nuclei in Brain Stem

- **Medulla**: IX–XII
- **Pons**: V–VIII
- **Mid Brain:** III, IV

Their corresponding symptoms and appropriate motor, sensory and reflex signs would accompany these.

Capsular Lesions

Capsular lesions are usually unilateral so do not produce a quadriparesis, unless there have been two separate lesions at different times. If so there will be a spastic quadriparesis with a pseudo-bulbar palsy (see page 131).

Cortical Lesions

To produce a quadriparesis at cortical level there have to be bilateral lesions involving both motor strips – these do not occur clinically.

Quadriparesis by frequency of occurrence

It is useful to consider causes of quadriparesis by frequency of occurrence and perhaps order of clinical importance, as advised for paraplegia. The list by probable frequency of occurrence which may vary with the age of the patient and country, is:

- Spinal cord compression
- AIDP of Guillain Barré type
- Cervical trauma
- Polyneuropathies
- Myopathies

- Neuronal disorders
- Myelitis.

HISTORY TAKING STATION

The requirements at the history taking station on quadriparesis are similar to those at the paraplegia history taking station (see pages 28–31).

As in paraplegia, a good history of the patient is invaluable in determining the nature and cause of the quadriplegia. Physical signs mainly help to localise the site of the lesion. At the end of the history the candidate must be able to draw a temporal profile of the quadriplegia (see Fig 14).

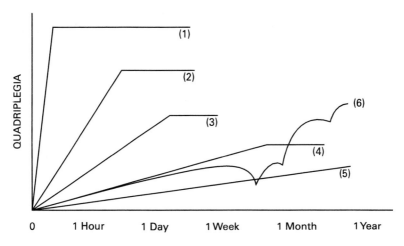

	Nature	Timescale	Condition/s
1	Ultra acute	Instant or minutes	Vertebral collapse, vascular
2	Acute	Within 24 hours	Polio, toxic, metabolic
3	Subacute	1–3 days	Epidural abscess
4	Progresses to plateau and improves	1–4 weeks for maximal deficit	Gullain Barré Transverse myelitis
5	'chronic' progressive	Months or years	Classical cord compression myopathy, degenerative disorders, neuropathies, some neuronal (MND)
6	Remittent or stepwise	Variable	Demyelination (MS)

Figure 14: Temporal profile of quadriplegia

It is also important to adopt a holistic approach towards the patient and ask them questions of ADL, as the patient may be quite disabled. As for paraplegia, the following specific points to be noted in the history include:

Time Frame

- Onset
- Progress
- Temporal profile
- Duration

This may fit in with the presentations shown in Fig 14.

Spatial Localisation

Motor

What is the distribution of weakness in the upper and lower limbs? Is the weakness global, proximal or distal? Is the weakness in the limbs symmetrical or asymmetrical? It may be possible to determine the nature of the gait by questioning (without examining, which is not allowed at the history taking station).

Is there any difficulty in walking? (See the paraplegia station, page 29.)

What is the patient's difficulty in using their arms – is it mainly weakness using the hand or is there difficulty at the shoulder also for common day-to-day tasks like combing or washing the hair?

Sensory

Ask specifically for pain and sensory disturbance.

Sphincter Disturbances

The bladder, bowel and sexual functions need to be assessed (see page 30). Having concentrated on the details of the quadriparesis, in the present complaint and its history, as in paraplegia, do not forget that there may be important clues from:

- Past history
- Family history
- Occupational history
- Social history
- Therapeutic history.

At the end of the 15 minutes of history taking, the candidate must be well prepared with the:

- Probable diagnosis with reasons
- Differential diagnosis
- Investigations
- Plan of management
- Résumé to be conveyed to the patient, relatives and GP.

FOOT DROP

NEUROLOGY STATION

A foot drop is apparent as a 'drop' or 'flop' of the anterior part of the foot and toes, on walking or standing on the heels.

During walking in a normal individual, the heel strikes the ground first, before the rest of the sole of the foot. In foot drop, the toes tend to scrape or 'stub' the ground when walking, making the person lift the foot higher, which produces a voluntary 'high stepping gait' on the affected side.

This is different to the high stepping gait seen bilaterally in peripheral neuropathy, which is due to a loss of sense of the position of the foot, in relation to the ground.

A foot drop is caused by **weakness of the dorsiflexors** of the foot and toes – anterior tibialis and peronei. A foot drop may be unilateral or bilateral. The weakness of the dorsiflexors may be due to lesions at either LMN or UMN levels. The former produces a flaccid foot drop with high stepping, while the latter produces a spastic foot drop where high stepping to clear the ground is not possible due to stiffness or spasticity.

First consider possible sites of the lesion which could produce a foot drop from an anatomical angle in a methodical manner. These sites are similar to those producing a paraplegia (see page 24).

Foot Drop – Sites of Lesion

SITE	DISEASE
Muscle	Myopathy
Neuromuscular junction	Myasthenia
Common peroneal nerve	Diabetes, Hansen's
Sciatic nerve	Trauma, Neurofibroma
Lumbosacral plexus	Pelvic pathology
L5 nerve root	L4/L5 disc prolapse
Cauda equina	Tumour

All above causes will produce a flaccid foot drop with LMN signs.

Flaccid Foot Drop

Consider sites and causes for localised weakness (see pages 7–23) and paraplegia (see page 24).

Muscle Level – Myopathies

As myopathies are proximal, foot drop is not often evident. However, there are exceptions to the rule – myopathies, which have a distal component like dystrophia myotonica (myotonia dystrophica).

In myotonia dystrophica, the foot drop is bilateral and symmetrical with an additional weakness of the foot – plantar flexion, inversion and eversion.

Other features include frontal balding, bilateral ptosis, cataracts, thyroid adenoma and gonadal atrophy. Look for myotonia where there is a slow or delayed relaxation after forceful voluntary contraction or percussion of the muscle.

Ask the patient to shake hands or grip your index and middle finger – there is a delayed relaxation of grip. Percussion myotonia can be found by tapping with the tendon hammer on thenar eminence, biceps, deltoid, quadriceps – a tapped portion forms a small bulge before disappearing slowly.

Percussion myotonia may also be elicited in the tongue. Tap on the tongue depressor placed on the tongue. The latter forms a dimple at the edge of the tongue depressor, which is known as a 'club sign' or 'trefoil sign' (the tongue takes the shape of a club – in a pack of cards).

Look also for the myotonic lid lag by asking the patient to follow your finger upwards and then slowly downwards – the upper eyelid lags behind the eyeball.

There are no sensory signs. Knee jerk (KJ) is often present but ankle jerk (AJ) may be absent.

Neuro-Muscular Junction – Myasthenia

Myasthenia presenting as an isolated foot drop is extremely rare. This is because isolated limb affection is uncommon.

If the foot drop is due to myasthenia it will have the hallmark of myasthenia – fatigability. The foot drop will appear with fatigue on walking or running. A foot drop that appears only on walking more often needs consideration of 'intermittent neurogenic claudication'.

If myasthenia is a possibility, look for fatigued ptosis, diplopia, dysarthria, dysphagia and proximal weakness, all of which may show fatigability.

Peroneal Nerve Palsy

Motor

The weakness of dorsiflexion of the foot is accompanied by weakness of eversion. In the rare deep branch of common peroneal nerve involvement, eversion is normal (see Fig 15).

Sensory

Sensation is affected in the outer lower leg and dorsum of the foot (see Fig 16). If only the deep peroneal branch is affected, sensory impairment is confined to the first inter-digital cleft.

Reflexes

Knee and ankle jerks are not affected.

The neck of the fibula is a common site for pressure palsy, which is more likely to occur when there is an underlying cause like diabetes, leprosy, collagenosis, alcoholic and other neuropathies.

The nerve can be palpated as it winds round the neck of the fibula by moving the finger vertically at the neck of the fibula. The nerve is thickened in Hansen's disease and some hereditary neuropathies like Dejerine and Sottas neuropathy.

Sciatic Nerve Palsy

Foot drop due to the sciatic nerve is uncommon. It may result from an incorrectly given intra-muscular gluteal injection (into the lower inner quadrant) or a neurofibroma. As well as the common peroneal nerve, the tibial nerve is also affected.

Motor

All muscles below the knee are weak, as well as knee flexion (hamstrings supplied by a branch of the sciatic nerve in the upper thigh). See Fig 17.

The following are not affected:

MOVEMENT	MUSCLE	NERVE	NERVE ROOT
Hip flexion	Ilio-psoas	N. to ilio-psoas	L1
Hip adduction	Adductors	Obturator	L2, 3,4
Hip extension	Glutei	Gluteal	L5, S1
Hip abduction	Glutei	Gluteal	L5, S1
Knee extension	Quadriceps	Femoral	L2, 3,4

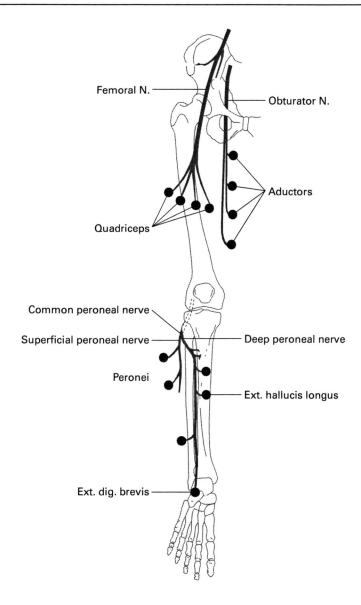

Figure 15: Femoral, obturator and peroneal nerves (modified from Aids to the Examination of the Peripheral Nervous System)

Sensory

There is more numbness than pain. Sensation is impaired in the back of the thigh and the whole of the lower leg, both anterior and posterior. See Fig 18.

Reflexes

AJ, plantar reflexes (S1) are absent or impaired.
Knee jerk supplied by the nerve to the quadriceps (L2, 3,4) is unimpaired.

Lumbosacral Plexus

Although uncommon, a unilateral lesion is produced by infiltrative lesions in the pelvis, which results in an excruciating ill-defined root pain. There is clinical evidence of multiple root lesions (see Fig 19). This is unlikely to be given in an examination.

L5 Root Lesion

Please note that the L5 nerve root arises from the L5 spinal level, opposite T12 vertebra (see Fig 5 as well as page 14 for revision). It has a long course from T12 to the lower border of L5 vertebra and then in the pelvis to form the lumbosacral plexus.

The most common cause is a L4/L5 disc prolapse. Others include neurofibroma and other cauda equina tumours.

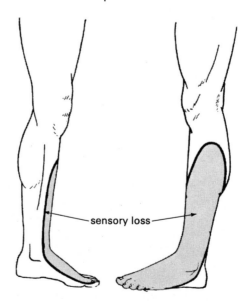

Figure 16: Sensory loss in common peroneal N (modified from Aids to the Examination of the Peripheral Nervous System)

L5 Root Pain

The root pain has a characteristic radiation.

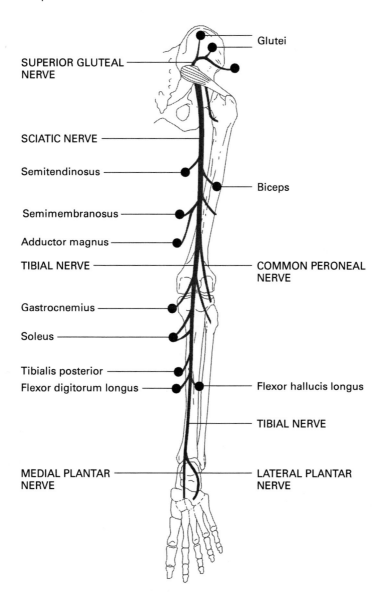

Figure 17: Sciatic Nerve and branches (modified from Aids and the Examination of the Peripheral Nervous System)

Lower back → buttocks → outer thigh → outer calf → dorsum of foot → big toe (and may include other toes except the little toe).

Motor

Weakness is limited to dorsiflexion of the foot and big toe only. A mild weakness of inversion may occur but there is no weakness of eversion which helps to differentiate it from a common peroneal nerve lesion. L4 and L5 roots also supply the tibialis posterior which invert the foot.

Sensory

This is similar to the common peroneal nerve but may extend to the outer thigh up to the buttock.

Reflexes

KJ, AJ and plantar are not affected. L5 supplies no reflex arcs.

Stretch Signs

The straight leg raising test may be positive – pain limits the movement.

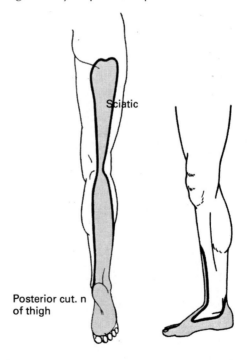

Sciatic

Posterior cut. n
of thigh

Figure 18: Sensory loss in sciatic nerve (modified from Aids to the Examination of the Peripheral Nervous System)

L5 Anterior Horn Cell (AHC)

The L5 anterior horn cell is situated in the spinal cord of L5 situated opposite the T12 vertebra. It was often due to poliomyelitis. It may also be caused by other diseases of the AHC, such as motor neurone disease and spinal muscular atrophy. Other features of the disease will be present.

Motor

This is the same as the L5 nerve root.

Sensory

No sensory impairment.

Reflexes

There is no abnormality.

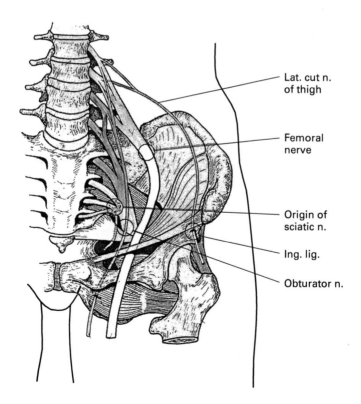

Lat. cut n. of thigh

Femoral nerve

Origin of sciatic n.

Ing. lig.

Obturator n.

Figure 19: Leg nerves in the pelvis

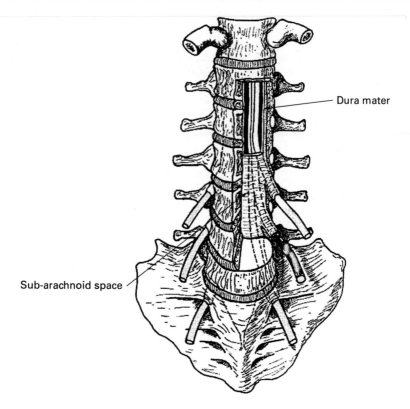

Dura mater

Sub-arachnoid space

Figure 20: Cauda Equina – Anterior view

Spastic Foot Drop

UMN weakness of dorsiflexors of the foot also produces a foot drop, which is usually not so apparent, as the spasticity does not allow the leg to be lifted, nor the foot to flop. In a high cauda equina lesion it is possible to have a foot drop with pyramidal signs.

Nevertheless, in hemiplegia the extensor hypertonia results in a spastic foot drop, which requires circumduction of the leg to clear the ground ('classical hemiplegic gait').

The spastic foot drop with a spastic weakness of the leg is often accompanied by weakness of the arm and a facial palsy. In bilateral spinal cord compression and parasagittal lesions, spasticity involves both legs and does not allow lifting of the feet or circumduction to compensate for the foot drop. This produces a spastic gait as though wading through mud or water.

HISTORY TAKING STATION

A relevant history could help in determining the site, nature and cause of lesion in many instances of foot drop – whether it is flaccid or spastic, unilateral or bilateral. After a careful history, it is often possible to have a reasonable idea of:

- **Site of lesion:** Spatial localisation
- **Nature of lesion:** Pathology
- **Cause:** Aetiology.

Useful Differential Points for a Flaccid Foot Drop

- Is it unilateral or bilateral?
- Is it symmetrical or asymmetrical?
- Is there a weakness other than dorsiflexion?
    - Plantar flexion
    - Eversion
    - Inversion
    - More proximal muscles
- Sensory symptoms and signs
- Disturbed physiology of micturition

Spatial Localisation of Foot Drop

Muscle Level

The only condition is myotonia dystrophica, so look for its diagnostic features – insidious, progressive, bilateral, symmetrical, floppy foot drop without sensory features or bladder involvement. The patient may complain about myotonia and gonadal atrophy upon direct questioning.

Neuromuscular Junction – Myasthenia

Unilateral or bilateral floppy foot drop only occurs on walking or running, and is associated with a myasthenic involvement of the eyelids, diplopia, dysarthria and dysphagia for liquids.

Common Peroneal Nerve

The floppy foot drop is associated with weakness of eversion and there may be sensory symptoms on the dorsum of the foot and outer calf.

Sciatic Nerve

The only direct trauma by injury or indirect trauma by intra-muscular injection or neurofibroma is responsible, the former being easily determined by the history.

Lumbosacral Plexus

Is there an excruciating pain indicative of a pelvic malignancy? Pelvic malignancy may affect the plexus or the pelvic part of the L5 nerve root.

L5 Lumbar Root

The patient often gives the classical radiation of pain described on page 14. Stretching the leg may worsen the pain and the patient may find it easier to sleep if they are turned to the opposite side with the affected leg flexed at the knee and hip. This may be accompanied by a complaint of a crooked spine (scoliosis) and ascending or descending sensory symptoms on standing or walking (neurogenic intermittent claudication).

The L5 root may be affected either in the pelvis (symptoms as above) or in the spinal canal. In the latter, ask the patient about symptoms of cauda equina involvement, particularly bladder symptoms and a numb perineum.

Cauda Equina Lesions

- **Low**: Involves only the nerve root – see the L5 root lesion mentioned in the L5 lumbar root section.
- **High**: Involves the L5 nerve root and possibly other nerve roots and a pyramidal tract.

L5 Motor Neurone

This used to be caused by polio. Now, although uncommon, it is due to motor neurone disease or spinal muscular atrophy.

Spastic Foot Drop

- **Bilateral**: In spinal cord compression.
- **Unilateral:** In hemiplegia.

Also see page 48 for features of spastic foot drop which need to be determined.

Nature of Foot Drop – Pathology

It is best to find out about the pathology of the site of the lesion.

Muscle Level – Myotonia Dystrophica

The patient may not complain or even be aware of the foot drop. The main complaints may be wasting of the muscles of the hand and neck or they could be related to myotonia. There will be a need to 'thaw' the 'frozen muscles' before embarking on an activity, e.g. exercise the limbs before getting up from a chair or getting into a vehicle.

Neuromuscular Junction – Myasthenia Gravis

This is very unlikely, as it is an extremely rare manifestation of myasthenia and only a theoretical possibility.

Common Peroneal Nerve Palsy

There are a few important common causes for a common peroneal nerve palsy:

- Pressure palsy is pressure at the neck of the fibula, which can happen when sleeping on a hard surface, especially after alcohol or restraining bands in the lithotomy position. Usually pressure on a nerve produces 'ischaemic paraesthesiae' and alerts the person to remove the pressure. This may not be present in a comatose individual or in diabetes with impaired post ischaemic paraesthesiae.
- Diabetes, alcohol abuse, leprosy and other causes of neuropathy need to be investigated.

Sciatic Nerve Palsy

- Trauma, often due to an intramuscular injection being given to the wrong quadrant of the buttocks – to the lower, inner quadrant instead of the upper outer one. It is rarely due to direct trauma, as the sciatic nerve is well protected by muscles and fat.
- Neurofibroma is uncommon but it is useful to ask for evidence of neurofibroma elsewhere. Look for café-au-lait spots and ask about family history.

Lumbosacral Plexus

This is rare and is usually due to an infiltrative lesion in the pelvis, which will produce excruciating pain in the lower abdomen, perineum and leg/s in root distribution. Ask the patient for other features of a malignancy of pelvic organs.

L5 Lumbar Root

- **L4/L5 lumbar disc prolapse**: Root pain in L5 distribution as it compresses L5 root.
- **Cauda equina lesion**: Root pain, bladder and sensory symptoms.

Causes of Foot Drop

The causes have already been dealt with in the section on the site and nature of the lesion (see page 40). It is useful to sum up the causes of foot by site and pathology.

Flaccid Foot Drop

SITE	DISORDER	ADDITIONAL FEATURES
Muscle	Myotonia	Autosomal dominant
NMJ	Myasthenia	Fatigability
Common peroneal N.	Mononeuropathy	Pressure palsy, other causes of neuropathy
Sciatic nerve	Neurofibroma	Incorrect IM injection
Pelvic plexus	Pelvic malignancy	Pelvic organ symptoms
L5 root in pelvis	Pelvic malignancy	
L5 root in spinal canal	Cauda equina tumour Disc prolapse	
High cauda equina	Tumour	Pyramidal signs
L5 Ant horn cell	Diseases of motor Neurone	Old polio, spinal muscular atrophy

Although it is theoretically possible for lesions in the spinal cord and brain stem to produce a foot drop, this is uncommon and unlikely to be an important facet of the clinical presentation. The most common cause of a spastic foot drop is a hemiplegia for unilateral (double hemiplegia if bilateral) and a parasagittal tumour for bilateral.

Spastic Foot Drop

SITE	DISORDER
Internal capsule	Stroke
Parasagittal	Tumour

HEMIPLEGIA

NEUROLOGY STATION

Hemiplegia is weakness of an arm and leg (usually of the same side) with or without facial weakness. The unilateral lesion is almost always UMN except on rare occasions with poliomyelitis. So myopathies, myasthenia, neuropathies, plexopathies, radiculopathies, neuronopathies do not apply to the differential diagnosis.

The UMN lesion is at brain stem, capsular, cortical or subcortical level. Rarely cervical lesions or hemi-parkinson's disease may mimic a hemiplegia. Look for other features of parkinsonism with TRAP:

T remor
R igidity
A kinesis or hypokinesis and bradykinesis
P ostural instability

See the flowcharts on page 64.

Descriptive terms

Crossed Hemiplegia

Crossed hemiplegia is a hemiplegia of one side with a contralateral LMN cranial nerve palsy, so may occur at mid brain, pontine or medullary level. The significance is that the lesion is at the level and the side of the cranial nerve palsy.

Recurrent Hemiplegia

This is recurrence of hemiplegia of the same side.

Double Hemiplegia

Hemiplegia of one side is followed by hemiplegia of the opposite side. It produces a quadriplegia, often asymmetrical, with or without a bulbar or a pseudo-bulbar palsy.

Site of Hemiplegia – Differential Signs for Localisation

The signs are elicited mainly to differentiate between a brain stem lesion and a capsular or cortical lesion. The presence and nature of a facial palsy is of utmost importance.

Facial Palsy

No Facial Palsy

The lesion may be mild and not affecting the fibres to the face. Or the site of the lesion does not have a facial representation as in:

1   cortical lesions not affecting the 'face area'
2   below pons:
   • **Medulla**: Cranial nerves IX–XII may be affected
   • **Cervical region:** Hemiplegia may rarely occur in cervical spondylosis
   • There may be some evidence of bilateral affection though the symptoms are unilateral. There may be evidence of long tract involvement of the unaffected side, i.e.:
      • Pyramidal: Brisk reflexes and extensor plantar
      • Spinothalamic: Loss of pain and temperature
      • Posterior column: Impaired position and vibration sense.

LMN Facial Palsy

The hemiparesis is on the side opposite the LMN facial palsy-crossed hemiplegia, and indicates that the lesion is at the level of the pons and on the side of the LMN facial palsy.

If the LMN facial palsy is on the same side as the hemiplegia, it means that the lesion in the pons is bilateral – one producing the facial palsy and the other the hemiplegia.

Other pontine cranial nerves may be affected – the Vth motor and the VI nerves, in particular (see Fig 9 on page 21 and see page 64 for flow diagram).

UMN Facial Palsy

The facial palsy would be on the same side as the hemiplegia i.e. it would be a face-arm-leg paralysis of one side. Sites of lesion could be:

• Mid brain
• Internal capsule
• Cerebral cortex.

Hemiplegia Due to a Mid Brain Lesion

The hemiplegia may be associated with:

• Contralateral III nerve palsy, i.e. a III nerve palsy of one side and a face-arm-leg paralysis of the opposite side – a crossed hemiplegia. This is Weber's syndrome (see Fig 11 on page 22) and is usually vascular.

- Ipsilateral cerebellar signs
- Loss of all modalities of sensation on the same side as the hemiplegia. (The spinothalamic tract and the posterior columns unite in the pons to form the medial leminiscus.) This also means that lesions above pons do not produce a dissociate sensory loss – there is loss of only some modalities – usually pain and temperature (see Fig 8 on page 21).

Hemiplegia Due to Capsular Lesion

The face-arm-leg paralysis may be accompanied by a hemi-anaesthesia or hemianopia (see Fig 12 on page 23).

Hemiplegia Due to Cortical and Subcortical Lesions

Useful differential features include:

- Conjugate deviation of eyes
- Speech defects
- Cortical sensory signs
- Parietal lobe signs.

Conjugate Deviation of the Eyes

This physical sign is particularly useful in differentiating a cortical lesion from a pontine lesion in the acute phase.

The pontine gaze centre controls the gaze to the same side, so a lesion of the pons will cause the head and eyes to move to the opposite side, i.e. to the paralysed side.

The frontal gaze centre controls the movement of head and eyes to the opposite side. So a cortical lesion will cause the head and eyes to move away from the paralysed side. (Irritative lesions of the frontal lobe like epileptic discharges will deviate the head and eyes to the opposite side as in the so-called 'adversive seizure'.)

To sum up:

- The pontine lesion moves the head and eyes to the paralysed side.
- The cortical lesion moves the head and eyes away from the paralysed side.

Visual Field Defects

The visual pathway does not cross the brain stem. So field defects are seen only with capsular and subcortical lesions. The field defect seen is usually a hemianopia on the same side as the hemiplegia in capsular and subcortical lesions. Look for visual inattention which may occur with parietal lobe lesions (see Fig 21).

Speech Defects

Is the speech:

- Normal?
- Dysphonic (hoarse)?
- Dysarthric (stutter)?
- Dysphasic (global, expressive, comprehensive, jargon, nominal or fluent)?

Brain stem lesions produce only a defect in articulation, producing a dysarthria or dysphonia.

Cortical lesions may produce a global or expressive dysphasia accompanying the hemiplegia when the dominant hemisphere is the site of pathology.

More posteriorly placed dominant hemisphere lesions may produce a receptive, fluent, jargon or nominal dysphasia without a hemiplegia. Sites of lesion for the speech abnormalities are:

- **Dysphasia:** Cortical
- **Dysarthria:** Brain stem or capsular
- **Dysphonia:** Medullary, posterior fossa, base of skull. Neck or thorax.

Cortical Sensory Loss

Cortical lesions (post central gyrus, Fig 22 on page 57) do not produce 'crude sensory loss'. A careful examination is needed to detect the following points on page 57, with the eyes closed.

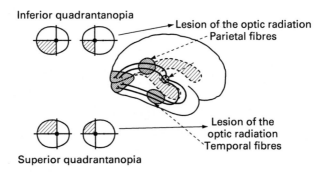

Figure 21: Field defects in cortical lesions

- 1 point discrimination
- Ability to differentiate texture, e.g. cotton and silk
- Localisation of touch and pain
- 2 point discrimination: Ability to differentiate whether the patient is touched with 1 point or 2 points placed 5 mm apart on the finger tips and 3 cm on the soles of shodden feet
- 3 point discrimination: Ability to tell the shape and size of objects, therefore identifying it with eyes closed
- Sensory inattention: Ability to appreciate simultaneous stimuli on identical sites of the two sides of the body.

Parietal Lobe Signs

With dominant parietal lobe lesions the following apply:

- Dyscalculia
- Dysgraphia
- Left/right disorientation
- Finger agnosia.

A combination of those four features constitutes the 'Gerstmann's syndrome':

- **Apraxia:** Inability to perform an act in the absence of weakness, incoordination or sensory loss.
- **Agnosia:** Inability to recognise an object in the presence of normal vision.

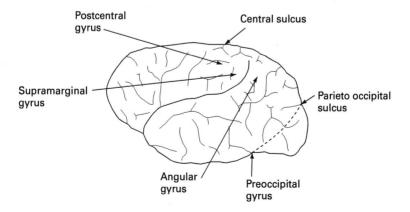

Figure 22: Parietal lobe

With non-dominant parietal lobe disease there is:

- Visual-spatial disorientation
- Constructional apraxia
- Dressing apraxia.

Features common to both parietal lobes include:

- Cortical sensory loss of the opposite side
- Contralateral lower quadrantic homonymous hemianopia
- Sensory and visual inattention of objects on opposite side.

Common Causes of Hemiplegia

Stroke

- Ischaemia in carotid circulation
- Ischaemia in vertebro-basilar circulation
- Cerebral haemorrhage
- Associated with subarachnoid haemorrhage
- Subdural haematoma

Mass Lesions (Space Occupying Lesions)

- Cerebral tumour
- Cerebral abscess

Hemi-Parkinson's Disease

- **Cerebral:** Irrespective of the site of lesion, the most common cause is a stroke – either ischaemia or a haemorrhage. This could be in the carotid or vertebro-basilar circulation, and it is almost always possible to determine which circulation is affected (see Fig 23 on cerebral circulation, page 59).

Cortical and capsular lesions: Carotid circulation

Brain stem lesions: Vertebro-basilar circulation

At cortical level, space occupying (SOL) or mass lesions like tumours, cerebral abscesses and subdural haematoma, need to be considered, especially when the onset is insidious or too slow for a vascular event or if it is progressive.

When the onset of the hemiparesis is over a few days, it is too slow for a vascular lesion and far too fast for a tumour. Two important conditions to be excluded are a cerebral abscess and a subdural haematoma.

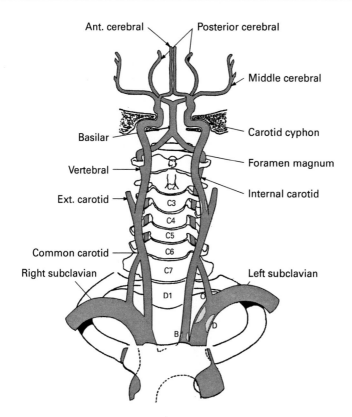

Ant. cerebral

Posterior cerebral

Middle cerebral

Carotid cyphon

Basilar

Foramen magnum

Vertebral

Internal carotid

Ext. carotid

C3

C4

C5

Common carotid

C6

Right subclavian

C7

Left subclavian

D1

Figure 23: Carotid and vertebral arteries

About 1% of acute hemiplegias suggestive of a vascular event may be due to an underlying mass lesion (see Fig 24).

In the initial phase of Parkinson's disease, the symptoms may be unilateral, shown as a mild to moderate weakness of one side (hemiparesis). Features of Parkinson's disease – tremor, rigidity, bradykinesis and postural instability must be looked for.

It is essential to be able to differentiate between a stroke in the carotid circulation from one in the vertebro-basilar circulation, particularly because those involving the cortex need the exclusion of space-occupying lesions.

Those in the carotid circulation may require further investigation, particularly imaging (CT or MRI) while those in the vertebrobasilar circulation are unlikely to harbour mass lesions. The investigations, prognosis and treatment may also differ.

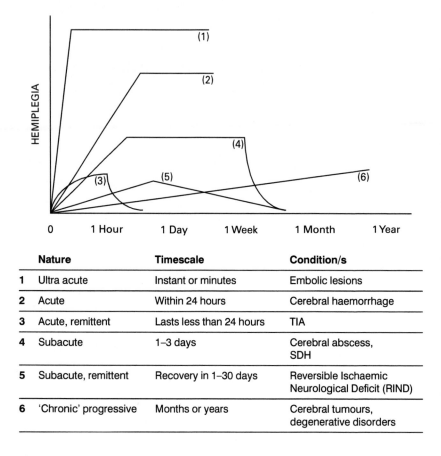

	Nature	Timescale	Condition/s
1	Ultra acute	Instant or minutes	Embolic lesions
2	Acute	Within 24 hours	Cerebral haemorrhage
3	Acute, remittent	Lasts less than 24 hours	TIA
4	Subacute	1–3 days	Cerebral abscess, SDH
5	Subacute, remittent	Recovery in 1–30 days	Reversible Ischaemic Neurological Deficit (RIND)
6	'Chronic' progressive	Months or years	Cerebral tumours, degenerative disorders

Figure 24: Temporal profile of hemiplegia

It is not so important to be able to differentiate between a middle cerebral and anterior cerebral stroke, though a knowledge of the areas of supply is important. Stenotic lesions in the common or internal carotid artery can embolise into either vessel.

Carotid vs Vertebro-Basilar Circulation

	CAROTID	VERTEBRO-BASILAR
Amaurosis	+/-	0
Diplopia	0	+/–
Speech	dysphasia	dysarthria
Vertigo	0	+/–
Ataxia	0	+/–
Facial	UMN	UMN in mid brain, contralateral
		LMN in pons, absent below pontine level
Other cranial N	0	LMN III – XII possible
Pyramidal	unilateral	may be bilateral
Bruits	carotid +/–	Vertebral +/–
		(supraclavicular fossa)

HISTORY TAKING STATION

The history in a patient with hemiplegia or hemiparesis should be taken with a view to the following.

Confirm the Hemiplegia

You have to establish that there is a weakness of the arm and leg on one side, with or without a facial palsy.

Determine the Severity of the Hemiplegia

Determine the severity of the weakness by noting how it affects ADL. Of particular importance are:

- **Walking:** Can the patient walk alone or do they need the assistance of a stick or the help of one or two individuals?
- **Talking:** Do they understand questions and answer rationally or is the speech slurred or hoarse?
- **Eating and swallowing:** Is there any difficulty in chewing and swallowing?
- **Bladder and bowel control:** Ask the patient about this.

It is also important to establish the deficit at the onset, particularly whether there was impairment of consciousness.

Onset and Progress of the Hemiplegia (Temporal Profile)

Two important aspects need to be determined:

- How long did it take for the maximal disability to appear?
- Has the weakness improved, worsened or remained static since the onset and in what way has it changed?

It should be possible to draw a graph to depict the temporal profile to differentiate a stroke from other common causes of hemiplegia (see Fig 24 on page 60).

To summarise, the hemiparesis usually happens:

- Within 24 hours – with a stroke
- In months or years with a tumour
- In 2–3 days with an SDH or cerebral abscess.

The temporal profile should enable the candidate to determine the cause or nature of the lesion.

Features (Symptoms) Accompanying the Hemiplegia

These features will help to find the site of the lesion and whether or not it is a hemisphere or a brain stem lesion. Impairment of consciousness may occur with either and is more indicative of the severity of the lesion.

Hemisphere Lesion

Symptoms include impairment of comprehension or expression, conjugate deviation of eyes away from the paralysed side, and a hemianopic field defect.

Brain Stem Lesion

Symptoms include diplopia, dysarthria, dysphonia, dysphagia, nasal regurgitation, checker board sensory impairment, ataxia and inco-ordination.

Features Determining the Underlying Cause

The following features may help in suggesting the underlying pathology.

Headache

Acute, severe occipito cervical headache occurs with Subarachnoid Haemorrhage (SAH). Continued awakening headaches with vomiting occurs in mass lesions with raised intracranial pressure.

Head Injury

This raises the possibility of Subdural Haematoma (SDH) and SAH.

Gait

While the'classical' circumducting gait may be seen after a stroke, the gait is more dragging in hemi-Parkinson's and functional hemiparesis.

Risk Factors

- **Family history:** Of stroke, cardiac or other vascular disease
- **Vascular risk factors:** Hypertension, diabetes, smoking, alcohol abuse, obesity, contraceptive pill
- **Cardiac pathology:** In favour of a stroke (particularly embolic)
- **Psychological trauma:** Functional hemiplegia

Features Useful for Prognosis

The prognosis depends on the cause or underlying pathology which can be deduced after the history. With a stroke, the prognosis also depends on:

- The age of the patient (worse after the age of 70 years)
- Level of consciousness at the time of maximal deficit
- Severity of the weakness
- Presence of dysphagia
- Incontinence and time for onset of and speed of recovery.

Investigations Carried Out

Most, if not all, patients would have had at least a **CT head scan** done. Some would have had an **MRI scan**, depending partly on the suspected pathology and partly on availability of the facility.

Other investigations would give a clue on the condition/s considered in the diagnosis:

- 2D Echo, Duplex carotid scan for cerebral infarct
- CSF examination: SAH, meningitis which may have resulted in an abscess
- Cerebral angiography: SAH.

Treatment Given

- **Surgical:** SDH, SAH due to an aneurysm or AVM, cerebral tumour, or cerebral abscess
- **Medical:** For hypertension, diabetes, and heart disease, aspirin, dipyridamole, anticoagulants. I.V. antibiotics for meningitis and cerebral abscess.
- **Psychiatric evaluation:** Functional hemiparesis.

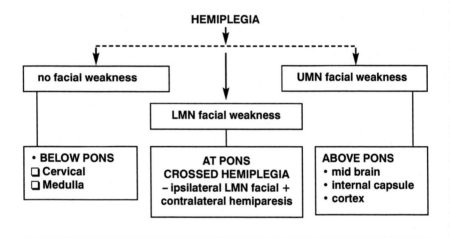

HEMIPLEGIA

| no facial weakness | LMN facial weakness | UMN facial weakness |

- **BELOW PONS**
  ❏ Cervical
  ❏ Medulla

AT PONS
CROSSED HEMIPLEGIA
– ipsilateral LMN facial +
contralateral hemiparesis

ABOVE PONS
- mid brain
- internal capsule
- cortex

LOCALISING SITE OF HEMIPLEGIA –
HELPFUL FEATURES
- **facial palsy** – see above
- **conjugate deviation of eyes**
- **visual field defects**
- **speech defects**
- **parietal lobe signs**
- **sensory signs**

WASTING/WEAKNESS OF SMALL MUSCLES OF HAND

NEUROLOGY STATION

As there is wasting of individual muscles, only LMN lesions need to be considered.

Sites and Causes of Wasting of Small Muscles of the Hand

MUSCLE	NERVE	N.ROOT	ACTION
Dorsal interossei	Ulnar n.	C8T1	Abduction (D–AB)
Palmar interossei	Ulnar n.	C8T1	Adduction (P–AD)
Abd. Pollicis brevis (APB)	Median n.	C8T1	Thumb abduction at right angle to palm
Opponens pollicis	Median n.	C8T1	Opposing thumb
Abductor digiti minimi	Ulnar n.	C8T1	Abduction of little finger

Muscle – Myopathy

Myopathies are generally proximal but exceptions include myotonia dystrophica and the rare distal myopathy (AD). Wasting is bilateral and symmetrical as in other myopathies and other features of myotonia dystrophica may be obvious. There are no sensory symptoms or signs.

Nerve – Ulnar, Median or Ulnar and Median

Ulnar Nerve

Ulnar nerve lesions produce wasting of dorsal interossei (guttering), hypothenar eminence, clawing of the little finger and partial clawing of the ring finger (see Fig 25).

Sensory impairment includes palmar and dorsal aspects of the little finger and the ulnar aspect of the ring finger and corresponding area of the hand. It does not extend above the wrist (see Fig 26 on page 67).

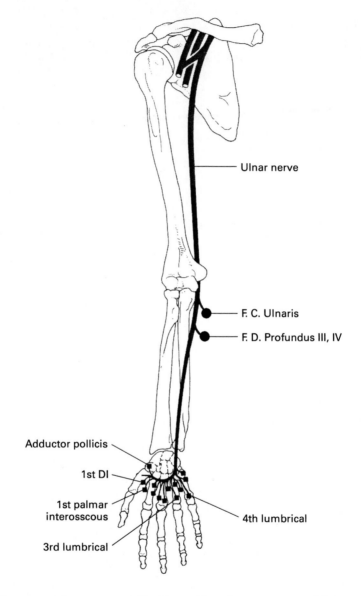

Figure 25: Ulnar nerve (modified from Aids to the Examination of the Peripheral Nervous System).

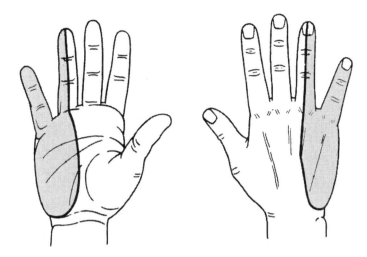

Figure 26: Ulnar sensory loss (modified from Aids to the Examination of the Peripheral Nervous System)

It is often due to a pressure palsy at the elbow, as seen in the cubital syndrome, due to an increased carrying angle with associated over-ride of the ulnar nerve over the medial epicondyle on flexing the elbow. Consider underlying diabetes, Hansen's and collagen disease.

Median Nerve

The abductor pollicis brevis (APB) is the only intrinsic muscle in the hand that is invariably supplied by the median nerve. (The opponens pollicis is often supplied by the median nerve – in about 90% of the population – see Fig 27.)

The most common lesion of the median nerve is evident in carpal tunnel syndrome (CTS). The sensory symptoms of numb fingers results from activities of a clenched fist, e.g. sewing, gripping, writing and may be worse at night.

Median nerve lesions produce:

- Wasting of the outer aspect of the thenar eminence (APB wasting)
- Weakness of abduction of the thumb at right angles to the palm (APB)
- Opposition of the thumb to the finger tips (opponens pollicis).

The sensory distribution of the median nerve is the thumb, index and middle fingers distally (Fig 28 on page 69) but may be more extensive in CTS.

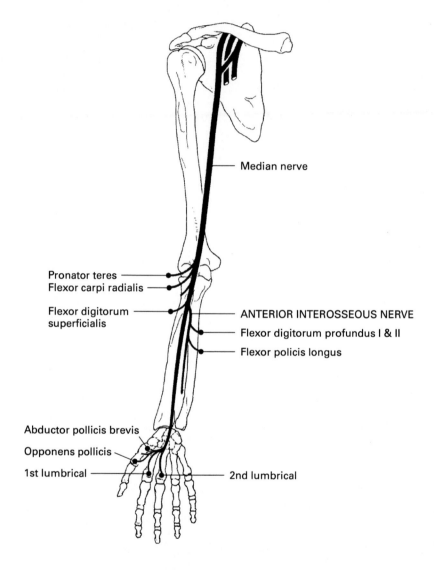

Figure 27: Median nerve (modified from Aids to the Examination of the Peripheral Nervous System)

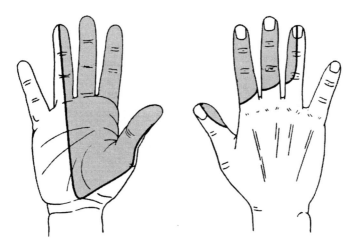

Figure 28: Median nerve sensory distribution (modified from Aids to the Examination of the Peripheral Nervous System)

Combined Ulnar and Median Nerve Lesions

These produce a true claw hand of all four fingers, with sensory impairment of the palm and all four fingers and thumb.

Lower Brachial Plexus Lesion – Thoracic Inlet Syndrome

Motor

This involves the muscles supplied by T1 nerve root, but often it may only be the APB that is affected.

Sensory

C8T1 distribution: There may be pain in the axilla, inner upper arm, inner aspect of the forearm and the ulnar aspect of the hand. The sensory impairment involves the inner aspect of the forearm in addition to the inner aspect of the palm, little finger and ulnar aspect of the ring finger (see Fig 29).

Vascular

The upward displacement of the brachial artery may lead to a diminished or absent brachial or radial pulsation. There may be stenosis with subsequent peripheral embolisation.

EMG

The EMG is very characteristic with the following.

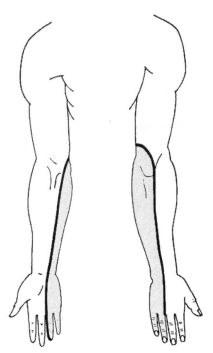

Figure 29: C8T1 sensory loss (modified from permission from Aids to the Examination of the Peripheral Nervous System)

- **APB:** Denervated with normal median nerve action potential
- **First dorsal interosseous**: Normal with absent action potential at the wrist.

C8T1 Cord Lesions

Motor

This mainly produces a weakness, with or without wasting, of APB, interossei, and hypothenar muscles.

Sensory

This does not apply as the neuronal pool is affected.

Causes

- **Motor Neurone Disease (MND):** Wasting of intrinsic muscles is a common early manifestation which could precede long tract and bulbar manifestations by a few years

- **Syringomyelia:** This occurs usually in young adults. They have a suspended dissociate sensory loss in the chest and arms (see Fig 30) with pyramidal signs in the legs (dissociate sensory loss – some modalities like pain and temperature are affected while others like position and vibration sense are unaffected).
- **Poliomyelitis:** This may be seen as a rare residual manifestation of old polio but rarely as an isolated manifestation
- **Distal Spinal Muscular Atrophy (DSMA):** This produces an asymmetrical wasting of intrinsics. It affects the forearm muscles (with spontaneous arrest in 3–7 years) without long tract signs in young adults in some Asian patients.

Note: Cervical spondylosis usually occurs at C5/C6 levels and is not a common cause of small muscle wasting.

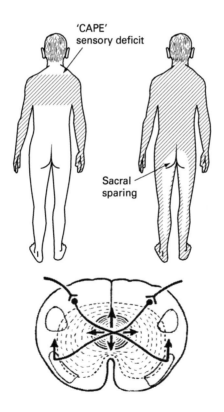

Figure 30: Sensory loss in intra-medullary lesions

HISTORY TAKING STATION

The aims in history taking are to:

- Determine the site and cause of lesion
- Determine investigations needed and carried out
- Plan management
- Prognosticate to the patient and relations.

Determine the Site and Cause

Onset and Progress

Small muscle wasting is always insidious but it can be noted incidentally, so may be thought to last only a short time. It is useful to know whether it is still progressive and whether it is now involving the other hand or ipsilateral forearm. The patient might not be able to say whether it is progressing with certainty.

Is it Unilateral or Bilateral?

UNILATERAL	BILATERAL
Neuropathy	Myopathy
Brachial plexus lesions	Neuropathy
	Neuronal lesions

Sensory Symptoms

- **Absent:** Myopathy, motor neuropathy, neuronal lesions
- **Fingers:** Neuropathy
- **Bilateral and dissociate:** Syringomyelia. Painless burns are a feature.

Other Manifestations

- **Myotonia:** Myotonia dystrophica.
- **Neuropathy:** Sensory motor disturbances elsewhere
- **Brachial plexus:** Root pains, vascular lesions
- **Spinal cord:** Involvement of legs and sphincters, fasciculation

Family History

Myotonia dystrophica is autosomal dominant.

Trauma

This is evident at the elbow, axilla, clavicle or cervical spine.

Occupation

Ask about occupations which may cause pressure on the ulnar nerve at the elbow.

Underlying Diseases

These include diabetes, Hansen's, collagen diseases and other causes of neuropathies.

Investigations Needed or Carried Out

As sites of lesions are at muscle and LMN levels, intracranial investigations are not indicated. Among the useful investigations are:

- **Blood:** CPK, aldolase, FBS, GTT, ESR, double strand DNA when indicated
- **CSF:** Usually normal and not of value
- **EMG and nerve conduction:** Very useful in most conditions, producing small muscle wasting
- **Imaging:** Plain films of the cervical spine and chest are mainly for a thoracic inlet syndrome. MRI of cervical spine, foramen magnum and posterior fossa are useful in intramedullary lesions like syringomyelia with craniospinal abnormalities.

Management

- Avoid trauma to the carpus, elbow, clavicle and neck
- Use surgery for carpal tunnel syndrome, cubital syndrome at elbow, thoracic inlet syndrome and syringomyelia
- Use physiotherapy for intrinsic muscles to improve the function and prevent contractures
- Drugs are not of much value

CLAW HAND

NEUROLOGY STATION

See the neurology station on wasting/weakness of small muscles of the hand on page 65) for sites and causes of the lesions, which are similar to the causes of small muscle wasting.

The Deformity

In a claw hand there is:

- Extension at the metacarpo-phalangeal joint (MCP)
- Flexion at the proximal interphalangeal joint (PIP)
- Flexion at the distal interphalangeal joint (DIP).

	MCP	PIP	DIP
Flexion	**Lumbricals**	Flexor digitorum	Flexor digitorum
	Interossei	Sublimis	Profundus
Extension	Extensor	**Lumbricals**	**Lumbricals**
	Digitorum	**Interossei**	**Interossei**

The deformity in a claw hand is the exact opposite of the functions of the interossei. So it could be said that a claw hand happens when there is a weakness of the lumbricals and interossei.

Or a claw hand could mean the weakness of lumbricals and interossei due to whatever cause.

Nerve Supply of Lumbricals and Interossei

MUSCLE	NERVE	NERVE ROOT
Dorsal interossei	Ulnar nerve	C8T1
Palmar interossei	Ulnar nerve	C8T1
Lumbricals		
Lateral two	Median nerve	C8T1
Medial two	Ulnar nerve	C8T1

Sites and Causes of Lesions

Not all conditions producing small muscle wasting will produce a claw hand. This is because there has to be a differential affection of the lumbricals and interossei with a preserved flexion at proximal and distal interphalangeal joints.

Only true LMN lesions from the lesions of nerve/s, brachial plexus, nerve root or C8T1 neurones can produce the highly localised wasting of lumbricals and interossei responsible for a claw hand.

- Nerve: Ulnar or ulnar + median nerve evident:
    - in the hand
    - at the wrist; or
    - forearm
    - elbow
    - upper arm
- Lower brachial plexus
- Nerve root
- C8T1 neurone pool

Ulnar Claw Hand

This only affects the little finger and partially the ring finger as the lateral two lumbricals supplied by the median nerve are not affected.

True Claw Hand

A true claw hand affects all the fingers except for the thumb. It is caused by a combined ulnar and median nerve or C8T1 lesions at the plexus, root or cord level.

Note: Solitary median nerve lesions only supply the lateral two lumbricals, APB and opponens pollicis, so do not produce a claw hand. The **hemiplegic hand** is not a claw hand. The hemiplegic hand is adducted and internally rotated at the shoulder, flexed and pronated at the elbow, flexed at the wrist and all the finger joints with adduction of the fingers. Also, a wrist and finger drop due to a radial nerve palsy does not produce a claw hand. However, there is apparent weakness of the interossei due to a lack of fixation at the wrist. To test interossei, the palm must be placed on a flat surface, especially when there is a wrist drop.

HISTORY TAKING STATION

This is similar to history taking for small muscle wasting (see page 72). Questions on myopathy do not apply.

WRIST DROP

NEUROLOGY STATION

Wrist drop is due to a weakness of extensors of the wrist – extensor digitorum, extensor indicis and extensor carpi ulnaris – all supplied by the radial nerve.

The posterior interosseous branch of the radial nerve (branching out in the forearm) supplies the extensors of the fingers, so the weakness invariably accompanies a wrist drop.

The radial nerve also supplies the brachioradialis, supinator and the triceps muscles. Examination for the weakness of these muscles helps to find the site of the lesion. The lesion is often located in the spiral groove in the posterior part of the middle of the humerus (see Fig 31).

Sites and Causes of Lesions

Lesions at the muscle and neuromuscular junction level are only theoretical possibilities.

Radial Nerve

Posterior Interosseous Nerve

This is rare and is usually compressed at the point of entry into the supinator muscle. It mainly produces a weakness of the extension of the thumb and index finger, with little or no wrist drop, and no affection of brachioradialis.

At the Spiral Groove

This is the most common lesion, caused by a pressure palsy in an inebriated, anaesthetised or unconscious patient. It produces a wrist and finger drop and also a weakness of the supinator (C5,6) and brachioradialis (C5,6).

In the Axilla

This is often caused by crutch trauma and sometimes by stab wounds and neoplastic involvement of axillary glands.

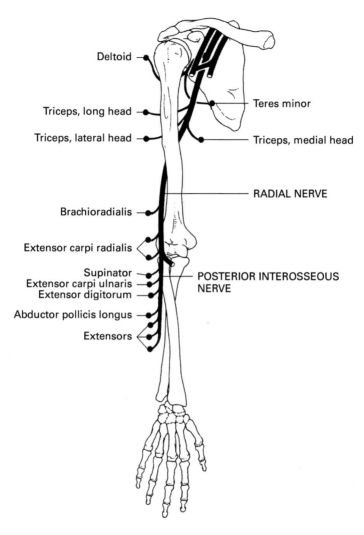

Figure 31: Axillary and radial nerves (modified from Aids to the Examination of the Peripheral Nervous System)

Motor

There is a weakness of the dorsiflexion of the wrist and extensors at the metacarpo-phalangeal joint. It is essential to examine the interossei with the palm on a flat surface to avoid non-existent weakness being detected by mistake.

Sensory

There may be a sensory impairment over the first dorsal interosseous space, dorsum of thumb and index finger but it is not common.

Brachial Plexus – Posterior Cord

This is essentially a radial nerve lesion combined with a circumflex nerve lesion. As well as the wrist drop there is a weakness of elbow extension and weakness of the second 90 degrees of shoulder abduction due to paralysis of the deltoid. This is often caused by bullet injuries.

Nerve Root

The C7 nerve root is responsible for the extension of the wrist. An isolated lesion of C7 is uncommon but it may be affected in cervical trauma and will indicate the level of lesion. It is rarely affected in cervical spondylosis.

Anterior Horn Cell

The isolated anterior horn cell disease of C7 could produce a wrist drop but this may be part of a more global weakness of the hand.

Traps

Mild Stroke

This may involve only the hand and could mimic a wrist drop.

Myotonia

In myotonia the slowness of relaxation may give the impression that there is a weakness of wrist extensors although there is no true wrist drop.

HISTORY TAKING STATION

Duration, Onset and Progress

Let the patient speak! In many instances the nature and cause of the wrist drop will become apparent. The specific questions that should be answered at the end of the history are:

- How long have you had this?
- How did it happen?
- Is it getting better, worse or static?

Trauma

Trauma is of particular importance with a wrist drop. At the spiral groove there will be pressure on the outstretched upper arm in an inebriated, unconscious or anaesthetised patient. It may also be caused by a fracture at this site.

The radial nerve can be compressed in the axilla by a crutch.

Injury to the cervical spine may be associated with a wrist drop but weakness of other muscles will be evident.

Additional Weakness

Is there a weakness of the brachioradialis and supinator? These are muscles which are supplied by the radial nerve. However, the nerve roots involved are C5 and C6 so they are not involved with the lower cord of the brachial plexus or lower cervical cord lesions.

Investigations

Usually this would be electrophysiological. If an MRI scan of the neck or axilla has been carried out it would mean the lesion is higher or more proximal.

Underlying Cause

The cause is often apparent from the history. Conditions which predispose to neuropathy like diabetes and collagen disease need to be excluded.

Management

Has it been a straightforward cockup splint and physiotherapy or have there been imaging procedures?

Prognosis

This depends on the underlying cause and the degree of improvement seen so far.

PROXIMAL MUSCLE WEAKNESS/WASTING

NEUROLOGY STATION

Not all conditions which produce shoulder wasting produce hip muscle wasting or weakness, so it is useful to consider them separately.

Weakness/Wasting of Shoulder Girdle

Shoulder girdle muscles include:

MUSCLE	NERVE	NERVE ROOT
Deltoid	Circumflex	C5,C6
Supraspinatus	Suprascapular	C5,C6
Infraspinatus	Suprascapular	C5,C6
Biceps	Musculocutaneous	C5,C6
Clav.pec.major	Medial pectoral	C5
Subscapularis	N to subscapularis	C5,C6
Serratus anterior	N to serratus ant.	C3,C4,C5
Latissimus dorsi	N to lat dorsi	C6,C7,C8

Sites and Causes

As for other localised wasting, sites and disorders are:

- **Muscle:** Myopathy
- **Nerve:** Neuropathy (uncommon)
- **Plexus:** Lateral cord
- **Root:** C5,C6
- **AHC:** C5,C6.

Useful Differential Points in Diagnosis

- Is it unilateral or bilateral?
- Is it symmetrical or asymmetrical?
- Is it painful or painless?
- What is the onset and duration?
- Is there a family history?

Bilateral Shoulder Weakness/Wasting

Symmetrical

This is usually apparent in myopathies. See the general features of myopathies (page 12). A useful simplified clinical classification is given here.

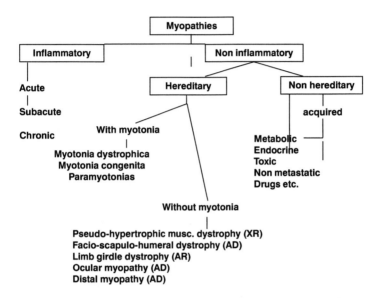

Inflammatory myopathies may be acute, subacute or chronic. Acute polymyositis may show features of inflammation – a red, hot, painful, swelling with loss of function. It is essential to look for an underlying cause such as collagen disease or malignancy elsewhere (commonly bronchus) particularly in the subacute, chronic and intermittent varieties.

Porphyria is the only common neuropathy to affect the proximal musculature.

Some of the conditions listed under asymmetrical wasting may sometimes be symmetrical.

Asymmetrical

Myasthenia

This can rarely present itself with a fatigable weakness of proximal muscles with remissions. After many years there may be symmetrical or asymmetrical wasting of the proximal muscles, at which stage fatigability might not be a feature.

Brachial Plexus Lesions

This is very rarely bilateral in sarcoidosis or traction injuries of the plexus. Muscles affected depend on the extent of plexus involvement.

Cervical Spondylosis

This is usually preceded by a C5 root pain, radiating from the side of the neck to the outer upper and forearm. It may be unilateral or rarely bilateral symmetrically or asymmetrically.

Proximal Spinal Muscular Atrophy (Kugelberg Welander Syndrome)

There is insidious progressive weakness and wasting without sensory manifestations. It may be mistaken for a muscular dystrophy especially when there is a family history – autosomal recessive (AR) and elevation of Creatine Phosphokinase (CPK). EMG is of great value in differentiation. It shows high voltage polymorphic waves (fasciculation potentials) often with fragmentation.

Unilateral Shoulder Weakness/Wasting

Peripheral Nerves

Of the peripheral nerves supplying the shoulder muscle only the circumflex and nerve to the serratus anterior are often affected. The former is affected with low intramuscular injections to the deltoid. Weakness of abduction of the shoulder is accompanied by a sensory impairment of a small longitudinally oval patch over the deltoid. Involvement of the nerve to the serratus anterior produces a winged scapula.

Brachial Plexus

Neuralgic Amyotrophy

This is the most common cause of unilateral proximal muscle wasting. There is usually a radicular pain beforehand which is often severe. Weakness of one or more of the C5,C6 innervated muscles follows. The deltoid, spinati, biceps, triceps and serratus anterior are usually affected. Slow recovery may take as long as one year.

Erb's Palsy

This is an avulsion of C5,C6 nerve roots by trauma – Road Traffic Accidents (RTA) or forceps delivery. The arm cannot be abducted at the shoulder and flexed at the elbow and hangs limply by the side. Though hand muscles are normal, it cannot be brought to a functional position.

Nerve Root

The C5 or C6 nerve root may be affected by a disc prolapse – acutely or chronically by a compressive lesion like a neurofibroma.

Motor

This is as described above.

Sensory

There is an impairment of sensation of the outer upper and forearm, thumb and index finger (see Fig 32).

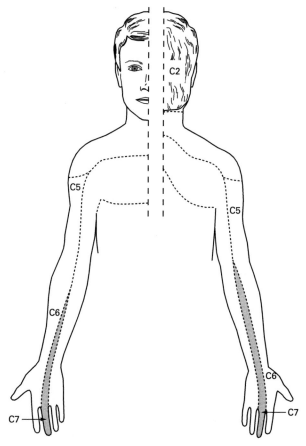

Figure 32: C5, C6 sensory loss

Reflex

There is a diminished or absent BJ and SJ.

Cervical Cord

There may be a diminished or absent BJ and SJ with a brisk TJ. The supinator jerk may be inverted.Intramedullary lesions are usually bilateral. Motor neurone disease may be considered a possibility.

Weakness and Wasting of Proximal Muscles of Lower Limbs

Proximal muscles of lower limbs include:

MUSCLE	NERVE	NERVE ROOT
Iliopsoas	N to iliopsoas	L1,2
Glutei	Gluteal nerves	L5,S1
Hip Adductors	Obturator N	L2,3,4
Hip Abductors	Gluteal N	L4,L5,S1
Quadriceps	Femoral N	L3,4
Hamstrings	N to hamstrings	L5,S1

Weakness of proximal musculature of the upper limbs is generally considered to involve the shoulder girdle muscles. Weakness of proximal musculature of the lower limbs is generally considered to involve the muscles of the hip and knees.

It is presented as a weakness of flexion at the hips and knees. Initially there is difficulty in getting up from a squat or low chair and climbing the stairs. Later the patient may have falls. There may be a waddling gait and lordosis.

Bilateral Weakness

Sites and causes are similar to bilateral weakness of shoulder muscles.

- **Myopathy:** See table above
- **Myasthenia:** Asymmetrical. This is a theoretical possibility.
- **Neuropathy:** Bilateral proximal neuropathy is unusual
- **Lumbosacral plexus lesions**: This is most common in pelvic malignancy
- **Proximal spinal muscular atrophy of Kugelberg and Welander**

Unilateral Weakness

This indicates either a root or nerve lesion (femoral or obturator nerve) and is often found in diabetic amyotrophy.

HISTORY TAKING STATION

Aspects to be considered are similar to other causes of localised wasting like small muscle wasting, claw hand, wrist drop, etc.

Duration, Onset And Progress

- **Myopathies:** Chronic and progressive
- **Myasthenia:** Intermittent with fatigue
- **Plexus and nerve root:** With pain and often unilateral
- **Neuronal:** Chronic and often progressive

Trauma

Trauma is of particular importance with acute unilateral lesions of the shoulder musculature. Injury to the cervical spine may be direct or more commonly indirect as in traffic accidents. Localised hip weakness is seldom due to trauma.

Additional Weakness

If the weakness is more than a localised proximal affection, it is unlikely to be a muscle or root lesion. With shoulder weakness, ask about spastic involvement of the legs to exclude a cervical cord lesion.

Investigations

Usually it would be electrophysiological. If myopathy is being considered a muscle biopsy may have been done. If there has been an MRI scan of the neck it would mean that a cervical cord lesion has been considered.

Management

Has surgery been offered as a treatment? Or has it only been physiotherapy analgesics and perhaps steroid therapy?

Prognosis

This depends on the underlying cause and the degree of improvement seen to date. Has the patient being made aware of the prognosis?

DIFFICULTY IN WALKING AND DISORDERS OF GAIT

NEUROLOGY STATION

Difficulty in Walking

Due to Weakness

- LMN
- UMN
- Foot drop
- Proximal muscle weakness

Read the sections on paraplegia (see pages 24–31), foot drop (see pages 40–52) and proximal lower limb weakness (see pages 84–85).

Due to Ataxia

- Cerebellar (see page 88)
- Sensory (see page 87)

Due to Rigidity and Bradykinesis

- Rigid akinetic syndromes

Vertigo

See pages 153–155.

Falls

See pages 178–181.

Apraxia

The difficulty is present in the absence of weakness, inco-ordination or sensory disturbance. Broadly the difficulty may arise from a defect in the conceptualisation (ideational) or conversion of the concept to the activity (ideo-motor).

Disorders of Gait

It is important to carefully observe the legs, hips, arm swing and eyes while the patient walks towards and away from you. It may be necessary to concentrate on one facet at a time. Also ask the patient to walk heel-toe in a straight line (tandem gait).

The gait is best carried out unshodden with legs well exposed. In a normal individual, during walking the heel touches the ground first, before the sole and toes. In foot drop the toes stub the ground and slippers tend to fall off. A patient with a foot drop cannot walk on his heels.

Muscle – Myopathy – Waddling Gait

Myopathies produce weakness of the spine and proximal muscles, a lordosis and a swing of the hips from side to side (waddle). Due to the proximal muscle weakness there will also be difficulty in getting up from a squatting position or a low chair and there will be a positive climbing up sign (Gower's sign). Myotonia dystrophica, however, produces symmetrical peripheral weakness and a bilateral flaccid foot drop.

NMJ – Myasthenia

The gait may be normal at the beginning but the patient may develop a flaccid foot drop or progressive difficulty as they continue to walk (with fatigue). This needs to be differentiated from a foot drop developing in neurogenic claudication, where there are often ascending or descending sensory symptoms in the legs on walking.

Nerve – Peroneal Nerve Palsy

This may be unilateral or bilateral, producing a flaccid or floppy foot drop. The feet are lifted high to clear the ground, producing a 'high stepping gait'. If there is sensory impairment as well, the patient often looks down at their feet. This is because the absence of position sense does not allow them to tell the distance of the foot from the ground, which may come down with a stamp (stamping gait).

Bilateral UMN – Spastic Gait

Both legs are spastic and cannot be lifted off the ground. The patient walks with stiff legs with hardly any flexion at the knees, as though wading through water or mud. The patient is unable to run.

Unilateral UMN or Hemiplegic Gait

There is unilateral spasticity with flexor hypertonia in the upper limb and extensor hypertonia in the leg. The arm is adducted and internally rotated at the shoulder, flexed and pronated at the elbow, flexed at the wrist and fingers.

The leg is stiff and extended at the knee and ankle and the patient tilts towards the opposite and circumducts the leg to clear the ground. Hemiplegics who recover early and well do not develop the 'classical hemiplegic gait'.

Scissor Gait

This is classically seen in cerebral palsy. The legs are stiff with adduction at the knees, resulting in the crossing of legs on walking and often at rest. In spite of the stiffness the patient may be able to walk quite fast, scissoring at the legs and walking on the toes, as they have adapted to the gait from childhood.

Cerebellar Gait

The patient walks with an unsteady gait with feet planted wide apart and arms outstretched to hold on to support and for equilibrium. The ataxia will be accentuated when walking with feet close together or heel toe walking (tandem gait). It is not made worse by closing the eyes. In patients with severe midline cerebellar disease producing truncal ataxia, the lack of balance may be seen even in the seated position.

Parkinsonian Gait

There is difficulty in initiation with several tentative starts, followed by a slow shuffle before patients accelerate and propel themselves, sometimes at a faster pace than a normal walk. Initiation is helped by lifting the foot off the ground.

Choreiform Gait

Movements of the arms and face produce a bizarre gait, likened to that of an oriental dancer.

Functional Gait

Any of the above gaits can be mimicked by an intelligent individual. A unilateral foot drag is the most popular but hemiplegic and reeling gaits are also common.

There could also be a combination of gaits.

Spastic Ataxic Gait

The spastic gait is modified by a super-added unsteadiness. This is when there is a combination of cerebellar and pyramidal signs, as may happen with cerebello-pontine angle lesions and lesions around the foramen magnum.

Recurrent falls may happen to patients with myoclonic epilepsy, drop attacks and SSPE (Subscute sclerosing panencephalitis).

Stance

The stance is best examined before the gait. Note the ability of the patient to stand with their feet together and also the ability to stand on their toes and heels. See whether there is any unsteadiness on closing the eyes – a positive Romberg's sign is evident in those with impaired position sense. The 'wash basin sign' is a manifestation of the Romberg's sign.

HISTORY TAKING STATION

The history aims to find out whether the difficulty in walking is due to a weakness, unsteadiness or other factors (see page 86). From the history it may be possible to determine the abnormality in gait and therefore the disorder and the cause. This will enable the candidate to prognosticate and advise on management.

INVOLUNTARY MOVEMENTS

INTRODUCTION

The most common involuntary movements to be found are:

- tremor
- chorea
- athetosis
- dystonia
- myoclonic jerks.

All involuntary movements except myoclonic jerks are absent or diminished during sleep and worsened by stress.

The involuntary movements of extrapyramidal disease has a spectrum of affection – from the resting tremor of parkinsonism at one end to dystonia at the other. Chorea and athetosis are at the middle of the range, with one merging into the other (choreo-athetosis).

Tremor

Physiological Tremor

It is a fine tremor, aggravated by stress, particularly seen with fine movement and when observed?

Benign Essential Tremor

This is a familial fine tremor which may be present at rest and made worse by movement, especially when observed or under stress. It may be improved by alcohol, beta blockers or benzodiazepines.

Thyrotoxic Tremor

This is an exaggerated physiological tremor. There is a fine tremor of hands which may be accompanied by other features of thyrotoxicosis. Such features are warm moist palms, exophthalmos with eye signs – lid retraction, lid lag, impaired convergence and upward gaze.

Parkinsonian Tremor

This is a slow, coarse, compound (biplanar or multi-planar) resting tremor which decreases with voluntary movement. Look for other features of parkinsonism such as hypokinesis, rigidity and postural instability.

Intention Tremor

This is classically seen with cerebellar disease. It may be unilateral or bilateral, and is seen well on performing the finger-nose co-ordination. It may be accompanied by other cerebellar features of hypotonia, past pointing, decomposition of movement, rebound phenomenon and dysdiadochokinesia. Cerebellar tremor is not affected by eye closure.

Red Nucleus Tremor

This is an uncontrollable jerking action which shows on attempt at movement and is present throughout the movement (action tremor). Hemiballismus is a severe bizarre unilateral movement occurring with lesions of the Corpus Lusyii.

Flapping Tremor

This is a coarse flapping movement of the wrist and fingers when arms are outstretched with hyperextended wrists. It is seen most commonly in the pre-coma phase of hepatic encephalopathy and rarely in renal, cardiac and respiratory failure.

Wing Beating Tremor

This is seen best with arms abducted at the shoulders with elbows flexed. It is characteristically seen in Wilson's disease, which needs to be considered in any type of involuntary movement.

Chorea

This is a fidgety movement without purpose, which is made to look purposive (quasi-purposive) by the sufferer to avoid embarrassment. The movement is sudden, jerky and consecutively non-repetitive. It involves the face producing frowning, grimacing, angular smiling) the tongue (thrombone tremor), and limbs.

It may be unilateral – hemichorea. Chorea may be seen with rheumatic fever with or without carditis, but usually not with arthritis or raised ESR. Pregnancy, the oral contraceptive pill, senility and Huntington's disease (autosomal dominant with dementia) may also produce chorea.

Athetosis

This is a writhing or 'corkscrew' type of movement of the entire limb, which may be confined to one side. It is due to extrapyramidal disease.

Dystonia

This is a severe distortional movement which may involve the trunk producing an arching of the spine with athetotic movement of the limbs.

Athetosis and dystonia are mostly seen in children with cerebral palsy, basal ganglia damage due to kernicterus or dystonia musculorum deformans.

Myoclonus

Myoclonus occurs as brief, shock-like muscle jerks and may be localised or rarely generalised.

Tics

Tics resemble myoclonus but differ in that they are repetitive, stereotyped and can be voluntarily suppressed. Typical tics involve the face (blinking, sniffing, lip smacking) or the upper arms and neck – shoulder shrugging with inclination of the neck.

Myoclonic Jerks

Myoclonic jerks or myoclonus are brief shock-like movements involving single or many muscle groups. It may be a normal phenomenon on falling asleep or waking. In patients with sleep epilepsy, they may persist up to an hour after waking up. Myoclonus may occur on a genetic basis and also after anoxic brain damage. Myoclonic jerks occur in severe metabolic disease, Creutzfeldt-Jacob disease and subacute sclerosing panencephalitis (SSPE).

NEUROLOGY STATION

Nature of involuntary movement

Is it:

- a tremor? If so, is it fine or coarse and only with certain postures or movements?
- chorea?

- athetosis?
- choreo-athetosis?
- dystonia?

Note the presence or change in the involuntary movement in the following positions of the hand:

- Resting on the knees or thighs – to see a resting tremor
- Outstretched – for a 'postural tremor'
- Outstretched with wrists dorsi-flexed
- Performing the finger-nose test – note whether the tremor appears only on movement or becomes worse or better
- Arms abducted at the shoulder and flexed at the elbow – for wing beating tremor.

Observation of the involuntary movement in these positions is particularly important for tremor.

Look for causes

The cause depends on the nature of the movement – tremor, chorea, athetosis or dystonia.

Tremor

Look for other features of:

- **Thyrotoxicosis:** Goitre, eye signs, warm moist palms, tachycardia
- **Parkinson's disease:** Rigidity, bradykinesis, postural instability
- **Cerebellar disease:** Ataxia, dysdiadochokinesia, past pointing, rebound phenomenon if the tremor is seen mainly on finger nose testing
- **Mid brain** affection if it is an action tremor: Ptosis, squint, diplopia and long tract signs
- **Liver dysfunction:** Hepatomegaly and jaundice if it is a flapping tremor
- **A Kayser-Fleischer ring:** A greenish ring at the corneo-scleral junction which is sometimes visible with a torch.

Chorea

Look for features of:

- Carditis – tachycardia, murmurs – particularly a mid diastolic murmur in the mitral area
- Evidence of dementia.

HISTORY TAKING STATION

At the history taking station with a patient having involuntary movements the following need to be determined:

- Duration
- How it was first noticed
- Whether it is mainly with stressful situations
- Medication before onset of movements
- Family history of similar affection
- Any change with alcohol intake
- Whether present in sleep.

History in relation to possible cause

- **Thyrotoxicosis:** Loss of weight, excessive sweating, loose stools, heat intolerance
- **Parkinson's disease:** Difficulty in sitting, standing, walking, turning, falls
- **Cerebral palsy:** Birth trauma, particularly if the patient is a child

MOTOR DISTURBANCES IN CRANIAL NERVE SUPPLY

PTOSIS

NEUROLOGY STATION

Degrees of Ptosis

Within the limits of human variation, usually the upper eyelid is about the level of the upper border of the cornea (see Fig 33).

- **Complete ptosis:** The upper eyelid covers the whole eye
- **Moderate:** The eyelid comes to the pupillary level
- **Severe:** The eyelid is below pupillary level
- **Mild:** A few mm of the upper cornea is covered

Congenital ptosis and Horner's syndrome produces only a mild ptosis, while severe and complete ptosis are seen with severe lesions of the III nerve.

Pathophysiology of Ptosis

Ptosis is due to weakness of elevators of the upper eyelid. The elevators of the upper eyelid are levator palpebrae superioris (LPS) and the Mullerian muscle supplied by the cervical sympathetic nerve. So, ptosis is a weakness of LPS or the Mullerian muscle.

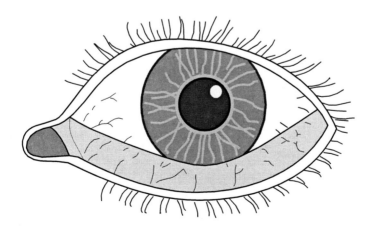

Figure 33: Eyelids in relation to cornea

Useful Differential Points for Diagnosis of Ptosis

- Duration and progress (old photographs are of immense value)
- Laterality
- Severity
- Presence of pain
- Diplopia
- Pupillary size and reaction
- Neighbouring cranial nerve symptoms and signs
- Family history
- Long tract signs

PTOSIS

Condition	Uni/bilat	Severity/ pain	Temporal profile	Family history	Diplopia	Pupils size	light	accom.	Other features
Horner's	unilateral	v. mild painless	variable	o	o	small Difficult to see	+	+	meiosis enopthalmos
Myopathy	bilateral symmet.	mod painless	v. slow progressive	+	0	normal			myotonia ± facioscap
Myasthenia	bilateral	variable painless	diurnal variation	0	+	normal (except cholinergic)			bulbar, limb
3rd nerve a) Orbital	unilateral	variable	progressive	0	+	variable			proptosis squint
b) Sup orb Fissure	unilateral	moderate painful	acute	0	+	normal			opthalmic sensory imp.
c) Cavernous sinus	uni/bil	severe painful	acute progressive	0	+	normal			chemosis, oph. max. sens. imp.
d) Post comm. aneurysm	unilateral	severe painful	acute	0	+	dilated	0	0	hypertensive elderly
Mid brain	uni>bil	moderate painless	variable	0	+	variable			long tract, pyr, extrapyr.
Congenital	uni/bilat	mild painless	static	+	0	normal			Marcus Gunn jaw winking ±
Tabes dorsalis	bilateral	mild painless	insidious static	0	0	small irregular	0	+	A incomp. AJ –
Migrainous neuralgia	unilateral	mild painful	acute	+	0	small regular	+	+	lacrimation conj. Injectin
Cranial Polyneuritis	uni/bilat	moderate	acute painful	0	+	normal			other CN ^ ESR ^ CSF protein

Sites of Lesion and Causes of Ptosis

Muscle – Ocular Myopathy

Myopathy of ocular muscles occurs in ocular myopathy (Autosomal Dominant AD), and in myotonia dystrophica (AD). There is insidious, slowly progressive, bilateral and symmetrical ptosis with external ophthalmoplegia. As ophthalmoplegia is symmetrical there is usually no diplopia.

Neuromuscular Junction – Myasthenia Gravis

This is the most common presentation of myasthenia. Often the ptosis is bilateral and asymmetrical with accompanying ptosis. There is often a history of varying severity of ptosis and diplopia. Ptosis alternating from one eye to the other is almost always due to myasthenia.

Fatigability can be demonstrated by repeated blinking or a continued upward gaze. Look also for fatigability of speech by asking the patient to count from 1–110. There is a difference in the quality of the 1–10 count and the 100–110 count. There may be dysphagia, nasal regurgitation and fatigable limb weakness.

Edrophonium ('Tensilon') Test

Edrophonium ('Tensilon') is available in 1 ml vials for intravenous use only. (1 ml=10mg). A test dose (0.2 ml = 2 mg) is first given and if there are no cholinergic effects, the remainder is given.

Improvement in ptosis, diplopia, speech, swallowing or limb weakness is noted. It is essential to decide which parameter is to be observed after the intravenous injection.

The test dose of Edrophonium is also used for:

- Differentiating a cholinergic crisis from a myasthenic crisis
- Noting adequacy of the dose of the cholinergic drug – by giving it one hour after oral neostigmine or two hours after oral pyridostigmine (time of maximal effect of drug).

Cholinergic Effects

Cholinergic effects are seen with an excess of an acetyl choline effect during treatment or with edrophonium, even with a test dose. Acetyl choline at the sites of action produces the following:

- **Neuro muscular junction:** Fasciculation
- **Sweat glands – (Cholinergic):** Excessive sweating.

At the parasympathetic endings of the cranial nerves:

- **III:** Constricted pupil
- **V,VII**: Excessive salivation and lacrimation
- **IX,X:** Bronchospasm and secretions, abdominal cramps and diarrhoea, bradycardia – occasionally cardiac arrest if edrophonium is given too rapidly to a sensitive subject.

Third (III) Nerve Palsy

In Orbit

Disorder has to affect the superior division of the III nerve supplying the LPS and the superior rectus muscles. Other nerves may be affected, producing a variable external ophthalmoplegia. There will be a downward proptosis.

Superior Orbital Fissure (SOF)

It is useful to remember the structures in SOF as **LFT SONIA** and the nerve supply as LR6 SO4, ie lateral rectus supplied by the VI nerve and superior oblique by the IV nerve and all others by the III nerve.

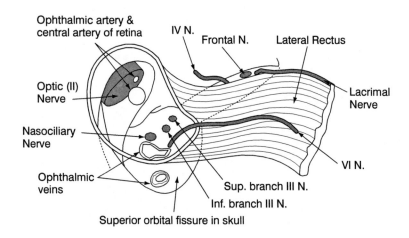

Figure 34: Third nerve in orbit and superior orbital fissure

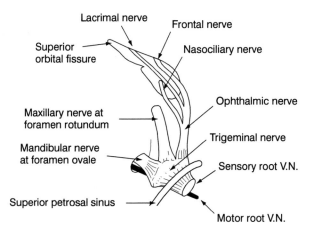

Figure 35: Superior Orbital Fissure and branches of v nerve

LFT SONIA stands for:

Lacrimal} Sensation in the opthalmic division
Frontal} of V
Trochlear: IV nerve supplying superior oblique muscle
Superior division of the oculomotor nerve
Ophthalmic veins
Nasociliary: Branch of ophthalmic V nerve including the nose. When vesicles appear in the distribution of this nerve in the ophthalmic zoster, there is a danger of affection of the cornea.
Inferior division of the oculomotor supplying the inferior rectus and inferior oblique.
Abducens: VI nerve supplying the lateral rectus.

The superior oblique is a depressor of the adducted eye. However, if the III nerve is paralysed, adduction is not possible. An attempt to look down produces internal rotation of the eye, when the IV nerve is intact in the presence of a III nerve palsy.

Cavernous Sinus

All structures finding their exit through the SOF are also found in the cavernous sinus. The cavernous sinus has one additional structure which exits through the foramen rotundum – maxillary branch of the V nerve (see Fig 36 on page 102).

So it is important to look for impaired sensation over the maxilla to differentiate a cavernous sinus lesion from an SOF lesion. Additional features with thrombosis of the cavernous sinus include proptosis, chemosis, conjunctival injection, engorged retinal veins and sometimes papilloedema.

Infranuclear

Posterior communicating aneurysm is the common lesion at this site producing an acute, painful, unilateral ptosis with a dilated pupil in an elderly hypertensive patient.

Mid Brain

In addition to the III nerve palsy, other structures affected include:

- **Pyramidal tract**: This produces a contralateral hemiparesis (crossed hemiplegia) also known as Weber's syndrome
- **Red nucleus**: Action tremor
- **Medial leminiscus**: Contralateral hemi-anaesthesia
- **Superior cerebellar peduncle**: Ipsilateral cerebellar signs
- **Superior colliculus**: Impaired upward gaze.

See Fig 8 on page 21.

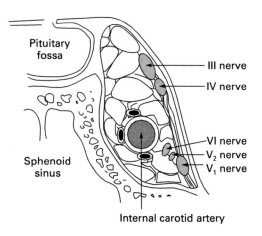

Figure 36: Cavernous sinus

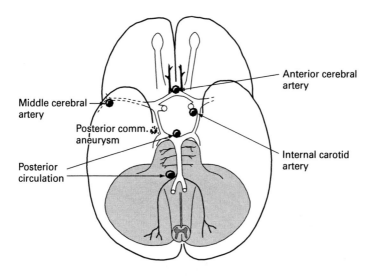

Figure 37: Posterior communicating aneurysm

Horner's Syndrome

This produces only a mild ptosis with only a partial coverage of the cornea by a few mm. Irrespective of the site and cause of the lesion the mild ptosis is accompanied by:

- **Meiosis (small pupil):** The pupil reacts to light and accommodation but the reaction may be difficult to note as the pupil is already small. The opposite reaction (dilation) is better seen when the eye is shaded or the patient looks far – this is the opposite of the usual technique for light and accommodation responses.
- **Enophthalmos:** This is the opposite of exophthalmos. The cornea is covered above by the upper eyelid and below by the lower eyelid.
- **Conjunctival injection:** This is due to a loss of vasoconstrictor activity.
- **Absence of sweating:** The area involved depends on the site of the lesion.

Sites of Lesions Producing Horner's Syndrome

Sympathetic pathway starts in hypothalamus, but clinically lesions are seen in the brain stem, cervical cord, T1 nerve root, neck and internal carotid artery – extra and intracranially (see Fig 38 on page 104).

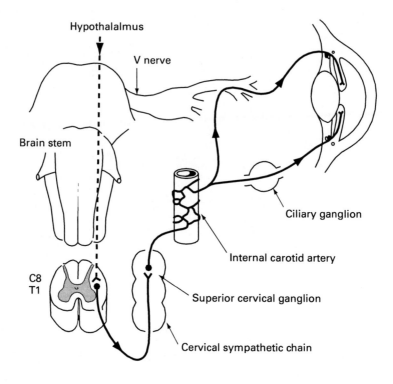

Figure 38: Sympathetic pathway

Brain Stem

Posterolateral lesions of the brain stem as in lateral medullary syndrome of Wallenberg, multiple sclerosis, brain stem encephalitis and pontine glioma, may produce a Horner's. It is often associated with contralateral hemi-anaesthesia due to proximity to the spinothalamic tract (see Fig 39 on page 105).

Cervical Cord

This is due to affection of the lateral column at T1 level. Pain and tempera-ture fibres around the central canal are also affected, producing dissociate sensory loss in the arms with hyporeflexia. Ptosis is mild and bilateral with symmetrical small reacting pupils.

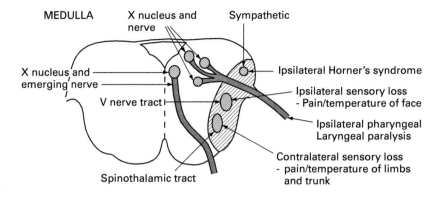

Figure 39: Lateral medullary syndrome

T1 Nerve Root

This is usually due to Pancoast's syndrome produced by an apical malignancy or thoracic outlet syndrome. C7/T1 disc prolapse is very rare.

Neck

Trauma, thyroid carcinoma and thyroid surgery, and malignant cervical lymphadenopathy are important common causes. Nasopharyngeal malignancy at the base of the skull may involve structures in the jugular foramen including cranial nerves IX–XI.

Carotid Artery

Lesions at this site may be seen in a migraine, internal carotid artery thrombosis, dissecting aneurysm of carotid and direct puncture of carotid.

The site of lesion is often apparent from the associated features. The area of impaired sweating could also localise the site of lesion. Lesions of the brain stem may impair sweating in the head, neck, arm and upper trunk of the same side.

The lower cervical region lesions impair sweating only in the face while lesions beyond the superior cervical ganglion do not impair sweating at all.

Others

See the Ptosis table on page 98. This includes congenital ptosis, tabes dorsalis and migrainous neuralgia.

HISTORY TAKING STATION

The history will, in most instances, be able to give an indication of the site, cause and nature of the lesion (see page 99).

Useful differential points are given on page 98.

The history will also give an indication of the investigations carried out, namely:

- Edrophonium test
- Electrophysiological studies
- Scanning – CT head, Ct thorax, MRI scan of head and chest
- Angiography if an aneurysm was suspected.

The advice given and treatment will indicate the prognosis and line of management contemplated.

PUPILLARY ABNORMALITIES

NEUROLOGY STATION

The size of the pupil is dependent on the interaction between the sympathetic and parasympathetic nerve activity. The parasympathetic nerve to the pupil is the III nerve.

Sympathetic **pupillodilator** activity is inherent and unaffected by external stimuli.

The degree of **pupilloconstrictor** activity of the III nerve is dependent on light stimulus through the optic nerve and light reflex pathway.

Sympathetic tone is less in infancy and old age, with a consequent physiologically small pupil at the extremes of age.

When there is more light → more optic nerve stimulation → greater III nerve stimulation → the pupil constricts.

Conversely the pupil dilates in the dark or in blindness, affecting the afferent light pathway.

A good light source is essential to note the size and pupillary reactions. It is not possible to observe the direct and consensual light reflex at the same time.

Small Reacting Pupils

- **Unilateral:** In Horner's syndrome
- **Bilateral:** In infancy and old age

Small Non-Reacting Pupils

- Instillation of pilocarpine or pupillary constrictor medication
- Opiate effect
- Pontine haemorrhage

Small Irregular Pupils

- **Iritis:** Small fixed pupils with no reaction to light or accommodation
- **Argyll Robertson pupil:** Small and eccentric, reacting to accommodation but not to light

Large Pupils

- **Unilateral:** Adie's pupil. A slow reacting pupil to light and accommodation (tonic pupil) may be associated with diminished reflexes.
- **Unilateral fixed dilated:** Compressive or III nerve palsy, mydriatics
- **Bilateral:** With normal reaction – anxiety due to pupillodilator sympathetic overactivity

Normal Size with Abnormal Reaction

An afferent pupillary defect is when there is no direct response but a consensual response is preserved. (If both optic nerves are severely affected and there is no perception of light, pupils will be dilated.)

PUPILLARY ABNORMALITIES

Condition	Uni/bilat	Diplopia	Visual impairment	Pupils Size	Light	Accommodation
Old, infants	bilateral	0	0	small	+	+
Holmes Adie's	unilateral	0	accom. difficult	large	slow (tonic) reaction	
Horner's	unilateral	0	0	small	+	+
Medical 3rd	unilateral	+	0		normal	
Surgical 3rd	unilateral	+	0	dilated	0	0
Argyll Robertson	uni/bilat	0 mild ptosis	0	small irregular	0	+
Iritis	uni/bilat	0	±	small irregular	0	0
Pontine hge	bilateral	0	0	small	difficult to see	
Cortical blindness	bilateral	0	+		normal	
Mydriatics	uni/bilat	0	accom. difficult	dilated	0	0
Pilocarpine	uni/bilat	0	+	small	difficult to see	

SQUINT AND DIPLOPIA

NEUROLOGY STATION

Squint

Squint is a deviation of one or both eyes, which may be:

- Unilateral or bilateral
- Convergent or divergent
- Congenital or acquired
- Paralytic or non-paralytic.

In congenital squint there is no ocular paresis (non-paralytic) and no diplopia. Weakness of abduction will produce a convergent squint, while weakness of adduction will produce a divergent one.

In an acquired squint due to acquired abduction or adduction palsy, vision may be normal, except for diplopia. In congenital squint, vision is often impaired in a squinting eye with suppression of its image and there is no diplopia.

Diplopia

(Also read the ptosis section on page 97.) In diplopia, there is an ocular paresis but this may not always be shown in ocular movements. There are a few useful rules connected with diplopia:

- Diplopia happens when the eyes are moved in the direction of the paralysed muscle action, e.g. on looking to the left with weakness of the left lateral rectus or right medial rectus
- False image is from the affected (paralysed) eye
- False image is the outer image even when there is no obvious ocular paresis. The affected eye can be determined by noting the eye from which the false image arises – the outer false image disappears on covering the affected eye (cover test).
- The image is tilted when there is affection of the oblique muscles – the superior is supplied by the IV or the inferior is supplied by the III. A lone VI palsy does not tilt the image.

Sites and Causes of Diplopia

Diplopia is produced by paresis of the oculomotor muscles supplied by the oculomotor nerves – III, IV, VI.

Muscle Level – Ocular Myopathy

In ocular myopathy, though extra-ocular muscles are markedly affected and there may be severe ptosis, the affection is symmetrical and there is usually no diplopia. There may be associated weakness of facial muscles with a 'transverse smile' and involvement of pharyngeal muscles with dysphagia.

In thyrotoxicosis, an inflammatory myopathic process may cause weakness of the superior and or lateral rectus.

NMJ – Myasthenia

Diplopia is common in myasthenia as the ocular muscle affection is often asymmetrical, including the ptosis. A continued gaze in the direction of diplopia may produce an increasing separation of images which indicate fatigability. There may or may not be associated bulbar and limb weakness.

Orbital Lesions

These may affect one or more of the oculomotor nerves and produce diplopia with ptosis and proptosis. The direction of diplopia and proptosis may indicate the location of orbital pathology. This is usually inflammatory, tumour or pseudo-tumour (orbital granuloma). Malignant infiltration of the orbit may result from carcinoma of the nasopharynx.

Superior Orbital Fissure

This may affect III,IV,VI cranial nerves as well as the ophthalmic V. Pain is an important feature. Usually there is no proptosis or affection of visual acuity.

Cavernous Sinus

Cavernous sinus thrombosis is still an important condition with painful ophthalmoplegia accompanied by conjunctival oedema, swelling of the lids and proptosis. It may become bilateral.

Often, the VI nerve is affected first. Intracavernous carotid aneurysms situated anteriorly could also produce a similar picture with associated blindness. If the aneurysm is more posteriorly situated it may produce pain over the ophthalmic V.

Rupture of the aneurysm would produce a carotico-cavernous fistula with a pulsating proptosis which may become bilateral. Such a fistula can arise from a fracture of the base of the skull with a tear of the carotid artery at the point of entry into a cavernous sinus.

At the Petrous Tip

Only the VI nerve is vulnerable at this site. This is often secondary to middle ear or mastoid infection. In addition to the VI, there may be associated VII and VIII affection (Gradenigo's syndrome). Mastoid infection may be associated with lateral sinus thrombosis and a rapid rise of intracarnial pressure. The VI nerve may also be affected at this site by spread of nasopharyngeal carcinoma.

Basal Lesions

An acute painful III nerve palsy with a dilated pupil may occur with a posterior communicating aneurysm. A giant aneurysm of the basilar artery could affect the III nerves bilaterally. The III nerve may also be affected by a prolapsing temporal lobe of a 'tentorial pressure cone' where a dilated pupil is followed by ptosis and a complete III palsy.

However, diplopia may not be a complaint as the patient is drowsy and ptosed. The VI nerve may also be affected in this region. This is particularly evident in children with a posterior fossa tumour. The dilated ventricles push down the brain stem, causing stretching of the VI nerves over the petrous tip.

All three oculomotor nerves may be affected by a basal meningeal infection – tuberculous, bacterial, carcinomatous or fungal. They are also rarely affected by sarcoid, maningovascular syphylis, or direct spread from a nasopharyngeal or paranasal carcinoma.

Brain Stem – Pons And Mid Brain

This is usually by vascular, infiltrative or demyelinating lesions:

- **Nuclear level**: Vascular and infiltrative lesions mainly
- **Inter-nuclear**: Classically with weakness of adducting eye, and nystagmus in abducting eye. Commonly in multiple sclerosis and less commonly in Wernicke's encephalopathy.

Note: MND does not affect oculomotor nuclei. Also UMN lesions do not produce diplopia or oculo paresis, but a gaze palsy.

HISTORY TAKING STATION

Also see ptosis on page 97.

To find out the cause of diplopia the following details are helpful:

- Onset – acute or progressive?
- Diurnal variation?
- Painful or painless?
- Cranial nerve/s affected?
- Proptosis, chemosis, conjunctival oedema?
- Evidence of raised intracrainial pressure and brain stem signs?
- Meningeal signs?
- Other symptoms of diabetes, thyrotoxicosis, multiple sclerosis?

NYSTAGMUS

NEUROLOGY STATION

Nystagmus is caused by a disorder of the ocular posture associated with a disorder of conjugate movement of the eyes.

A nystagmoid jerk is not a mild nystagmus. It is a coarse, jerky movement observed when the physical sign is elicited in the wrong way – the object is too close and moved too far and too fast! The candidate should therefore not use the term nystagmoid as it means that they are eliciting a false physical sign.

So it should **not** be given as a physical sign.

Differential points include:

- Is it fine or coarse?
- Is it present at rest?
- Direction of the gaze producing nystagmus – is it upward, downward or horizontal?
- Is it sustained or not?
- Direction of fast component – is it horizontal, vertical or rotatory?

Types

Congenital Nystagmus (Pendular)

Very obvious continuous nystagmus is present at rest and worsened by a gaze in any direction. It is a side to side movement without a fast component. It is often familial but can also be seen in retinal disease and coal miners. There is no accompanying vertigo and the patient is unaware of eye oscillation or oscillation of image (oscillopsia). The head may move in the opposite direction and the nystagmus remains horizontal on a vertical gaze.

Vestibular Nystagmus

There is often associated tinnitus, deafness or vertigo. Nystagmus is greater on looking to the side away from the lesion. It may be:

- **Peripheral**: At semicircular canals or the vestibular component of the VIII nerve
- **Central**: Vestibular nuclei in pons.

	PERIPHERAL	CENTRAL
Direction	Horizontal	Vertical
	Rotatory	Rotatory
Gaze	Conjugate	Dysconjugate ±
Vertigo	±	0
Continued gaze	Adapts	Persists
Visual fixation	Increases	No change
Causes	Labyrinthitis	MS, basilar isch
	Meniere's	Syringobulbia
	Alcohol	Glioma
	Middle ear disorders	

In vertical nystagmus eyes move up and down mainly on the upward gaze. It is often seen with brain stem disease but may also be observed with drug toxicity (phenytoin). Downbeat nystagmus on the horizontal gaze is almost pathognomonic of the lesions at the craniospinal junction.

Ataxic nystagmus or dissociate nystagmus is present when both eyes show different degrees of disturbed ocular posture. This usually manifests with nystagmus of greater amplitude and frequency in the abducting eye rather than the adducting eye. It is usually seen in multiple sclerosis with affection of the medial longitudinal bundle.

Cerebellar Nystagmus

This is greater on looking at the side of the lesion. Otherwise features are similar to central vestibular nystagmus. In midline cerebellar and degenerative cerebellar disease there may be severe ataxia and cerebellar signs without nystagmus. The nystagmus is often coarse. The exact mechanism is not quite clear.

Drug-induced Nystagmus

This can be seen in the use of anti-convulsants and alcohol.

HISTORY TAKING STATION

It is unlikely that a patient with nystagmus will be given for history taking, as it is a physical sign and only rarely produces the symptom of oscillopsia – a jerking of an image.

It is useful to know whether the abnormal movement has been noticed by the parents during childhood and whether the patient is aware of abnormal movements of the eyes. The drug history and whether there is accompanying tinnitus, deafness, vertigo or ataxia would be helpful in differentiating a labyrinthine from a cerebellar cause.

CONJUGATE GAZE PALSIES

NEUROLOGY STATION

Exact pathways of gaze control are complicated and are not totally under-stood, but for clinical purposes it is useful to consider three 'centres' connected with horizontal gaze.

Horizontal Gaze Centres

Frontal Gaze Centre
Stimulation of this centre causes head and eyes to move in the opposite direction. This is also under voluntary control.

Parieto-Occipital Gaze Centre
This is important for pursuit and visual fixation.

Pontine Gaze Centre
Stimulation produces movement of the head and eyes in the same direction.

Vertical Gaze Centres

This appears to be at mid brain level beneath the colliculi with some control by basal ganglia.

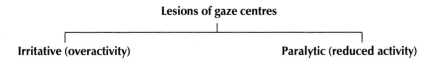

Lesions of gaze centres

Irritative (overactivity) Paralytic (reduced activity)

Irritative Lesions of Conjugate Gaze

Overactivity
This is usually due to seizures originating from the particular area, resulting in a partial or focal seizure, which may become generalised. (This is a secondary generalised seizure.) The spasm of gaze is seen at the onset of the

epileptiform attack and occasionally may be the only manifestation in an abortive attack.

Adversive Seizures (Originating from the Frontal Eye Fields)

The head and eyes move to the side opposite the affected irritative frontal lobe. This is followed by convulsive movements of the opposite side which may end in a generalised tonic clonic seizure.

Seizure Originating from Parieto-Occipital Cortex

The head and eyes deviate to the opposite side, followed by a generalised seizure. There may be an aura of visual hallucinations but as the motor area is at a distance there is no focal limb movement before the generalised seizure.

Oculogyric Crisis

This is produced by overactivity of the vertical gaze centres in the mid brain. It usually happens following phenothiazines and postencephalitic Parkinsonism.

Paralytic Lesions of Gaze – Gaze Palsies

Lesions of Frontal Eye Fields

Paralytic lesions of the frontal eye fields are mainly due to vascular lesions and will produce a **weakness** of the conjugate gaze to the opposite (paralysed) side. So the head and eyes will deviate **away** from the paralysed side. This may return to normal after several hours or occasionally days.

Parieto-Occipital Eye Fields

There is a weakness in pursuit movement. This may be difficult to test because of:

- An associated deficit in comprehension
- The homonymous hemianopia which accompanies vascular lesions which are often responsible.

It also produces a loss of opto-kinetic nystagmus.

Horizontal Gaze Centre

The pontine gaze centre is responsible for movement of the head and eyes to the same side. So pontine lesions will produce a paralysis of movement to the same side. These will therefore deviate to the opposite side, which is also the paralysed side.

There may be an associated ipsilateral VI nerve palsy with contralateral hemiplegia producing a crossed hemiplegia.

So in hemiplegia, the deviation of head and eyes helps to localise the lesion, whether it is cortical or pontine.

- **Pontine:** Eyes deviated to the **paralysed** side
- **Frontal:** Head and eyes to the non-paralysed side

The pontine gaze centre may be paralysed in ischaemic lesions in the vertebro-basilar territory and infiltrative lesions like pontine glioma.

Vertical Gaze Centre

Paralytic lesions of the vertical gaze centre may occur in old people, in multiple sclerosis, pinealoma, Wernicke's encephalopathy and neurosyphilis.

In the supranuclear palsy of Steele Richardson syndrome, there is a weakness of vertical gaze with Parkinsonian features and pseudo-bulbar palsy.

- **Superior collicular level:** Weakness of upward gaze with dilated non-reacting pupils
- **Inferior colliculus:** Impaired downward gaze, loss of convergence with normal light reflex

Medial Longitudinal Bundle (MLB)

The MLB is a longitudinal bundle running bilaterally from the mid brain to the pons connecting the III, IV, VI nerves to each other and its opposite number. It ensures smooth synchronised or conjugate movement of eyes.

A lesion here produces the following.

Classical Internuclear Ophthalmoplegia

There is a weakness of adduction with mild nystagmus on the lateral gaze while the abducting eye moves normally and shows obvious nystagmus **(ataxic or dissociate nystagmus).**

A bilateral lesion is classically seen in multiple sclerosis, while a unilateral lesion may occur with a unilateral brain stem ischaemia.

Other Internuclear Ophthalmoplegia

Divergent Squint

There is a paralysis of the medial recti producing a divergent squint bilaterally which may be accompanied by skew deviation and see-saw nystagmus. It occurs in multiple sclerosis and vascular lesions.

117

Convergent Squint

There is weakness of abduction of both eyes while adduction is normal, during horizontal conjugate movements. It is similar to a bilateral VI nerve palsy but eyes abduct independently when each eye is covered. As in classical internuclear opthalmoplegia, there is nystagmus in the abducting eye and there may be diplopia and blurring of vision.

HISTORY TAKING STATION

As conjugate palsy is unaccompanied by symptoms the patient will be unaware of its presence. It is unlikely that a person with a pure conjugate palsy will be given at the history taking station.

FACIAL PALSY

NEUROLOGY STATION

Sites of LMN Lesions

Muscle Level – Myopathy

Myopathies which affect the facial muscles will produce a symmetrical bilateral facial palsy. This includes facio-scapulo-humeral dystrophy and myotonia dystrophica.

NMJ – Myasthenia Gravis

It is unusual for myasthenia to show facial weakness but the latter can be found in diagnosed generalised myasthenia.

Facial Nerve

There are several sites of possible affection – LMN and UMN.

Sites of LMN affection

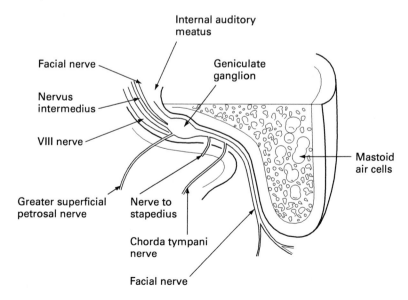

Figure 40: Facial nerve

- **Stylo-mastoid foramen:** This is seen with mixed parotid tumour.
- **Facial canal:** This is often found in Bell's palsy – all facial muscles are affected. However, during recovery the frontalis and orbicularis oculi may recover first, giving the false impression of lower facial muscle weakness only, mimicking a UMN facial palsy. When the affection is proximal to the union of chorda tympani branch, taste to the anterior 2/3 of the tongue may be affected. When it is proximal to the nerve to the stapedius muscle the patient may complain of hyperacusis.
- **Geniculate Ganglion:** This usually occurs with Herpes zoster infection (Ramsay Hunt syndrome). There may be preceding pain and herpetic vesicles in the external auditory meatus, auricle and mastoid area. There may be sensory symptoms in V and IX distribution.
- **Internal auditory meatus:** An acoustic neuroma at this site would have preceding auditory manifestaions – tinnitus and deafness.
- **Cerebello-pontine angle:** Initial symptoms are auditory – tinnitus and deafness. Vertigo is uncommon and LMN facial palsy is late. Impairment of the corneal reflex occurs before cerebello-pontine manifestations (with ipsilateral cerebellar and bilateral pyramidal signs). Raised intracranial pressure with headache and papilloedema is late.
- **Pons:** Depending on the extent and site of lesion, in addition to the LMN VII palsy, there may be:
  - Ipsilateral V palsy
  - Ipsilateral VI palsy
  - Ipsilateral VIII palsy
  - Weakness of conjugate gaze to side of lesion.
  - A crossed hemiplegia
  - Contralateral hemi-anaesthesia
  - Contralateral impairment of posterior column sensation.

Sites of UMN Lesions

Also read hemiplegia – mid brain, internal capsule and cortex on page 54.

Common Causes of Unilateral Facial Palsy

- Bell's palsy
- Local – trauma – history of base of skull fracture with bleeding from ear and mixed parotid tumour
- Middle ear disease
- Ramsay Hunt syndrome
- Cerebello-pontine angle lesions
- Pontine lesions
- Vertebro-basilar ischaemia at pontine level

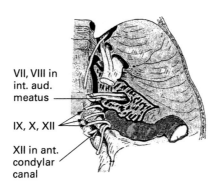

Figure 41: Cerebello-Pontine angle

Causes of Bilateral Facial Palsy

- Myopathies
- Guillain Barré syndrome
- Sarcoidosis

Causes of Cerebello-Pontine Angle Lesions

- Acoustic neuroma
- Meningioma
- Metastasis
- Cholesteatoma
- Aneurysm of basilar artery
- Rarely pontine glioma, astrocytoma and medullopblastoma in children

HISTORY TAKING STATION

The aim of the history station is to find out the following:

- Site and causes of lesion
- Investigations carried out
- Prognosis
- Treatment.

Sites and Causes of Lesions

- Is it unilateral or bilateral?
- Are the upper facial muscles – orbicularis oculi and frontalis – affected?
- What is the onset and progress?
- What are the associated symptoms:
  - Taste affection
  - Hyperacusis
  - Lacrimation
  - Tinnitus
  - Deafness
  - Vesicles in and around ear
  - Vertigo
  - Ataxia
  - Headache?

Investigations Carried Out

- Audiogram
- Imaging – plain films, CT, MRI
- Electrophysiology
- Cardio-vascular investigations – 2 Decho, duplex scanning

Prognosis

This depends on the recovery already made and the likely cause.

Management

Management will depend on the cause or likely cause. Physiotherapy is likely to have started, whatever the cause.

PALATAL PALSY, NASAL VOICE, AND NASAL REGURGITATION

NEUROLOGY STATION

The muscles of the palate are supplied by the vagus nerve (X). (The IX nerve is mainly sensory. The only motor supply of the IX nerve is to the clinically inconsequential stylopharyngeus muscle.) The main symptom is nasal regurgitation with nasal voice. X nerve affection also produces dysarthria, dysphonia and dysphagia.

Sites of palatal palsy

Muscle

This occurs in the rare oculo-pharyngeal myopathy.

Neuromuscular Junction – Myasthenia

This is not an uncommon symptom in myasthenics with bulbar involvement.

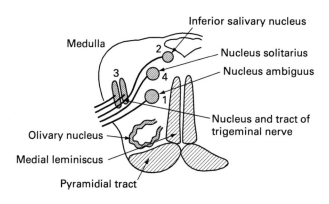

Figure 42: IXth nerve

Nerve

- In neck
- Nasopharynx
- Jugular foramen
- Basal meninges
- Posterior fossa
- Medulla

IX,X,XI nerves traverse the jugular foramen while the XII nerve exits through the anterior condylar foramen (see Fig 43).

Medulla

The most common cause of X nerve affection in the medulla is ischaemic – the lateral medullary syndrome of Wallenberg.

UMN Lesions

As there is bilateral representation of the X nerve for clinical manifestations to occur lesion has to be bilateral as in pseudo-bulbar palsy – see page 131.

HISTORY TAKING STATION

As in all conditions described it is important to attempt to localise the site of lesion from the extent of spatial involvement. Then the cause needs to be determined by defining the temporal profile.

Temporal Profile

This is done by determining the duration, onset and progress of the symptom.

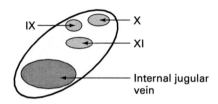

Figure 43: Jugular foramen

Spatial Localisation

This is done mainly by determining the accompanying symptoms, which in this instance would include the following:

- Extent of X nerve involvement – ask about dysarthria, dysphonia, dysphagia
- Involvement of neighbouring cranial nerves in:
  - brain stem – IX – pharyngeal sensation
  - XI – sterno-mastoid and trapezius
  - posterior fossa – VII – facial palsy
  - VIII – tinnitus, deafness, vertigo
  - jugular foramen – IX,XI
  - nasopharynx – V,XII
- Other structures in brain stem:
  - long tracts
    - pyramidal
    - posterior column
    - spinothalamic
  - cerebellar signs
  - Horner's
- UMN symptoms of pseudo-bulbar palsy – emotional incontinence in addition to dysarthria and dysphagia

Determining Specific Disorders

- Family history for myopathies
- Fatigability for myasthenia
- Causes of common neuropathies – diabetes

DYSARTHRIA AND DYSPHONIA

NEUROLOGY STATION

Dysarthria

Dysarthria is a disorder of articulation. Dysphonia is a defect in phonation, articulation being normal. The muscles of articulation are:

MUSCLE	CRANIAL NERVE
Jaw muscles	V
Lips, face	VII
Palate, pharynx, larynx	X
Tongue	XII

One or more of these muscles must be affected to produce dysarthria. This could be at the LMN or UMN level. Dysphonia is due to faulty adduction of vocal cords (X).

LMN Causes of Dysarthria

Muscle Level – Myopathies

Dysarthria is seen with the myopathies – in facio-scapulo-humeral and myotonia dystrophica dysarthria is mild, and not a presenting symptom.

NMJ – Myasthenia

Fatigable dysarthria with or without other features of myasthenia – fatiguable ptosis, diplopia, dysphagia and limb weakness.

Cranial Nerve Level

Lesions of V, VII, X, XII. These cranial nerves may be affected at the following levels:

- **Neck:** Any of the above cranial nerves
- **Nasopharynx:** Any of the above cranial nerves
- **Basal cranial foramina**

126

- **V:** Foramen lacerum
- **VII:** Internal auditory meatus (IAM)
- **X**: Jugular foramen
- **XII:** Anterior condylar foramen
- **Basal meninges**
- **Cranial fossae**
  - Middle fossa: V
  - Posterior fossa: VII,X,XII.

See Figs 44 and 45.

Brain Stem

- **V, VII:** Pons
- **X, XII:** Medulla

Inflammatory and malignant disease are common to all of the above sites. Additional causes are at:

- **Nerve level:** Diabetes, collagen vascular disease, sarcoidosis and cranial arteritis
- **Foramina:** Paget's disease
- **Brain stem:** Motor neurone disease, syringobulbia, bulbar polio, ischaemia and haemorrhage

UMN Causes of Dysarthria

Usually unilateral UMN lesions only affect the lower half of the face on the contralateral side. Even severe lesions produce only a mild dysarthria. So for

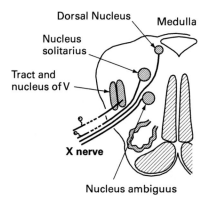

Figure 44: X nerve in medulla

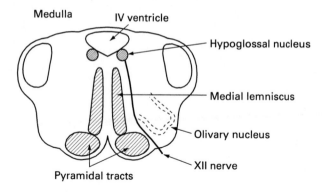

Figure 45: XII in medulla

V, VII, X, XII cranial nerves to be effectively involved at the UMN level, the lesion has to be bilateral. This usually happens with motor neurone disease (MND) and bilateral strokes (double hemiplegia) – see pseudo-bulbar palsy – on page 131.

Cerebellar Causes of Dysarthria

The articulatory muscles may be malfunctioning due to a lack of co-ordination in cerebellar disease. It could be unilateral or bilateral. It produces a staccato or explosive speech.

Extrapyramidal Causes of Dysarthria

Articulatory muscles may be affected by the slowness (bradykinesis) and poverty (hypokinesis) of movement in extrapyramidal disease, to produce a low volume festinant speech where words tend to tumble over one another. Dysphagia from neurological causes may also be due to disorders at the same level as those causing dysarthria.

Dysphonia

Dysphonia is produced by unilateral or bilateral vocal cord palsy. Speech is soft, hoarse or husky. It usually occurs with paresis of the vocal cords or palate. Palatal palsy produces a nasal speech. See causes under palatal palsy, on page 123.

Apart from causes listed under dysarthria, dysphonia may also be produced by lesions of the recurrent laryngeal nerve. The left recurrent laryngeal nerve may be damaged by an aneurysm of the aorta as the nerve winds round it.

Local causes of vocal cord involvement by acute or chronic laryngitis, TB and carcinoma are common non-neurological causes of dysphonia.

Hysterical dysphonia is not uncommon where articulation including lip movement is preserved but the voice is a whisper. The vocal cords adduct well as seen by a normal cough and at laryngoscopy.

HISTORY TAKING STATION

This is similar to the history for nasal regurgitation and palatal palsy (see page 124).

Keep in mind the causes by site of lesion, as given in the neurology station on palatal palsy (see page 123).

- Muscle – myopathies – oculopharyngeal and facio-scapulo humeral dystrophy
- Myasthenia
- Cranial neuropathies – also consider cranial polyneuritis
- Lesions in the neck, nasopharynx and base of skull
- Jugular foramen lesions
- Medullary lesions – particularly basilar iscaemia, MND, myasthenia
- UMN – pseudo-bulbar palsy – ischaemia or MND
- Cerebellar dysarthria
- Extrapyramidal disorders

BULBAR PALSY

NEUROLOGY STATION

The bulb is the brain stem and LMN or UMN lesions of the brain stem cause bulbar palsies. If the lesion is in the medulla and pons itself affecting the lower cranial nerves (V-XII), it is a **true bulbar pulsy**.

If the brain stem effect is secondary to bilateral UMN lesions of the brain stem it produces a **pseudo-bulbar palsy.** Both produce the combination of symptoms of dysarthria with dysphagia, but one has the features of LMN lesions and the other UMN features. The mid brain with its oculomotor nuclei is not usually affected in bulbar palsies.

BULBAR PALSY

Dysphagia + Dysarthria

	TRUE (LMN)	PSEUDO (UMN)
Tongue wasting	+	0
Tongue spasticity	0	+
Tongue fasciculation	+	0
Gag reflex	0	+
Jaw Jerk	0	++
Emotional incontinence	0	+

Levels of Bulbar Palsy and Causes

Muscle – Myopathic Bulbar Palsy

Usually mild as the pharynx is only mildly affected. It occurs in facio-scapulo-humeral, myotonia dystrophica and oculopharyngeal myopathies.

NMJ – Myasthenic Bulbar Palsy

This may be a manifestation of generalised myasthenia or can present acutely like an ischaemic bulbar palsy.

Neuropathic – Lower Cranial Nerve

Cranial nerves V, VII, X, XII may be affected in the neck, nasopharynx or base of the skull (also read the section on dysarthria on page 126).

Pons and Medulla – True Bulbar Palsy

This affects cranial nerve nuclei V, VII, X, XII in the pons and medulla. The causes are:

- Motor neurone disease
- Basilar ischaemia
- Brain stem glioma
- Syringobulbia
- Bulbar polio.

UMN – Pseudo-bulbar Palsy

Unilateral UMN lesions can produce a mild pseudo-bulbar palsy but the full blown picture is seen with bilateral lesions. The unilateral lesions may be mild and short lasting.

Bilateral UMN lesions may occur with motor neurone disease and with bilateral strokes.

Also, the bulbar muscles might not function properly due to:

- Affection of co-ordinated movement by involuntary movements
- Cerebellar disease
- By hypokinesis in extrapyramidal disorders, notably Parkinson's disease.

HISTORY TAKING STATION

The history in palatal palsy, dysarthria and bulbar palsy have features in common and may also be considered together as the sites of lesions and conditions producing them are similar.

Sites and Causes of Lesions

Nature of symptom/s

Which of the symptoms are present – nasal regurgitation, dysarthria, dysphagia?

- **Dysarthria**: Nature. Is a stutter present throughout articulation or is there fatigability, a tendency to be explosive or festination?

Dysphagia: At the onset was the dysphagia mainly for liquids or solids and which is more affected now?

Associated Symptoms

Is there any evidence of other cranial nerves being involved? Notably:

- **VII:** Facial palsy?
- **VIII:** Tinnitus, deafness and vertigo?

Evidence of Features of Causative Disease

Of particular importance would be vascular disease, motor neurone disease, syringomyelia and myasthenia.

Prognosis and Management

This depends on the cause, which may be apparent from the history.

WEAKNESS/WASTING OF THE TONGUE

NEUROLOGY STATION

The muscles of the tongue are supplied by the XII nerve originating in the medulla, traversing the posterior fossa and exiting through the anterior condylar foramen into the upper neck. Weakness of the tongue of one side causes it to deviate to the paralysed or wasted side, which is also the side of the lesion.

LMN lesions

- **Medulla:** Often occur in motor neurone disease. May also arise in syringobulbia, intrinsic tumours and extrinsic tumours in the region of the foramen magnum.
- **Posterior fossa:** May involve neighbouring IX, X, XI cranial nerves in the jugular foramen
- **Craniospinal junction:** With spinal cord long tract, medullary and cerebellar signs
- **Nasopharynx**
- **Neck**

UMN Lesions

The tongue has bilateral cortical representation so is not affected by unilateral UMN lesions. Bilateral UMN lesions produce a small spastic tongue seen classically in pseudo-bulbar palsy.

HISTORY TAKING STATION

The history taking under palatal palsy, nasal regurgitation, dysarthria, bulbar palsy is applicable to the wasting of the tongue (see page 124).

DISORDERS OF SPECIALISED FUNCTION

DISORDERS OF SPEECH

Clinically consider three possibilities:

- Dysphasia
- Dysarthria
- Dysphonia.

Dysarthria and dysphonia have already been dealt with (see page 126).

NEUROLOGY STATION

The cortical area for speech (dominant hemisphere) is in the left hemisphere in right-handed people.

Left-handed people may have speech and language function mainly on the right, or mainly on the left or shared between both sides.

Though speech centres are no longer recognised, expressive dysphasia occurs with anteriorly placed lesions and receptive dysphasia in posteriorly placed lesions of the 'dominant hemisphere'.

Expressive Dysphasia

(Anterior or Broca's aphasia.)

Comprehension of the spoken and written word is normal. Expression is poor with impaired non-fluent speech.

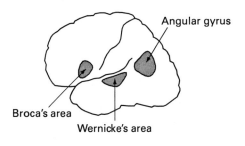

Figure 46: Speech areas

Receptive Dysphasia

(Posterior or Wernicke's dysphasia.)

There is difficulty in understanding the spoken and written word, while speech may be fluent and grammatical with normal articulation. However, it may lack meaning with inappropriate words or phrases (paraphasia) or new words (neologism).

Conduction Dysphasia

Lesions in the Perisylvian region may have elements of both expressive and receptive dysphasia. A characteristic feature is the difficulty in repeating heard speech.

HISTORY TAKING STATION

Onset and Progress

The onset and progress enables the candidate to tell the difference between a vascular lesion and an expanding mass lesion. It must be possible to determine the temporal profile of the deficit from the history.

The patient must be examined for the following aspects of speech.

Analysis of Speech Deficit

Understanding the Spoken Word

This is done by giving a complex verbal command, e.g. "When I lift my hand, not before, you close your eyes".

The patient should not be deaf. Asking them to put their tongue out is not a good question as this is a primitive survival reflex which the patient may do without any understanding.

Understanding the Written Word

Give a command in writing. The patient's vision must be intact.

Expression by the Spoken Word

Let the patient speak about the illness.

Expression by the Written Word

Obtain further details about the history of the illness in writing.

Reading

Difficulty in reading is termed dyslexia.

Spelling

Difficulty in spelling often accompanies dyslexia.

Other aspects of speech deficit to be checked include:

- Repeating
- Writing a dictated statement
- Copying
- Naming objects (nominal dysphasia)
- Parietal lobe dysfunction.

Look for dominant parietal lobe signs and those common to both the dominant and non-dominant hemisphere (see page 57).

In particular look for dysgraphia (writing difficulty), dyslexia (reading difficulty), dyscalculia and finger agnosia – the components of Gerstmann's syndrome.

Prognosis and Management

The prognosis depends partly on the underlying cause. Recovery from speech deficits is usually slow and may take many months and be incomplete. In addition to treatment of the cause, speech and language therapy is needed from a qualified speech therapist.

DISORDERS OF VISION

NEUROLOGY STATION

It is important to realise that when both eyes are open (binocular vision), there is considerable overlap between the fields of the two eyes. The main central field of vision is common to both eyes and a person could go blind in one eye without realising it, especially if the blindness is gradual. (This can easily be checked by looking straight ahead and closing one eye – only a small sector of the unimportant peripheral vision disappears.)

This also means that it is not possible to state the duration or onset of blindness, when the blindness in one eye is discovered incidentally or accidentally – either on closing of one eye or at examination.

Also, when a patient complains of impaired vision on one side, it is probably not due to impaired vision in that eye but due to a homonymous field defect on that side. A left homonymous hemianopia means that the left half of the visual field is not seen. This is not due to disease of the left eye but to a lesion in the right visual pathway.

Impaired Visual Acuity

Any patient complaining of impaired vision or others in whom the vision may be impaired, should have the visual acuity assessed by the following:

Snellen Chart

This is for assessing distant vision. With progressive impairment of distant vision, the deterioration of visual acuity can be quantitatively recorded as:

6/6 → 6/60 → 1/60 → counting fingers (CF) → finger movements (FM) → perception of light (PL) → no perception of light (NPL).

It is important to have serial assessment of visual acuity in patients with impaired vision as progressive visual loss requires energetic treatment to prevent blindness.

Reading Chart – N or J Chart

Serial quantitative assessment is again of importance in suspected progressive lesions.

Conditions impairing vision and visual acuity include:

- Corneal disease
- Lental opacification
- Abnormalities of refractory media
- Retinal disease
- Disease of the macula
- Optic nerve lesion
- Cortical lesions affecting macular vision.

Common conditions found which clinically produce impaired vision and visual acuity include:

- Optic neuritis (papillitis)
- Optic atrophy (primary and secondary)
- Hypertensive and diabetic retinopathy
- Central retinal artery occlusion
- Macular disease.

All these conditions are detected by examining the ocular fundi.

Ocular Fundi

It is important to master the examination of the ocular fundi by utilising the correct technique. Important details to follow are:

- For examination of the patient's right eye, the candidates should have the ophthalmoscope in their right hand and examine with their right eye – correspondingly for the left eye
- The patient is asked to fix their gaze on an object on the ceiling or wall with the other eye – slightly upwards and outwards
- When examining the eye the candidates should not allow their head to go across the midline of the patient's face – if they do, the patient's vision will be covered by the candidates' head and the pupils will constrict and hinder fundus examination.

The ocular fundi must be examined carefully for the five Cs.

C ontour of the disc
C olour of the disc
C up – of optic disc
C irculation
C uriosities

Contour is usually well demarcated but is blurred in papilloedema starting on the nasal side.

Colour of the disc is pink – pale in optic atrophy, more pink in optic neuritis and papilloedema.

Cup – clearly seen centrally as a pale white area. Larger in glaucoma, absent in papilloedema.

Circulation – vein/artery ratio of the retinal circulation is 3:2 in normal individuals, but veins are engorged with the onset of papilloedema. To note venous engorgement, occlusion of arterial branches and retinal veins it is useful to follow the vessels along the four main branches – superior nasal and temporal, inferior nasal and temporal.

Curiosities – macula, haemorrhages, exudates, pigmentation. There are two ways of visualising the macula:

- Visualise the optic disc and and tilt the ophthalmoscope slightly (two discs) temporally
- Ask the patient to fix the gaze on the ophthalmoscope light after reducing the aperture to prevent over-constriction of the pupil.

See the table on page 149 which should enable the candidate to tell the difference between papilloedema, optic neuritis (papillitis), primary and secondary optic atrophy.

The fundal appearance of papilloedema and optic neuritis may be very similar but differentiation is extremely important, and dependent on other features.

	PAPILLOEDEMA	OPTIC NEURITIS
Visual symptoms	May be absent	Always present
	'Amaurosis fugax'	Scotoma, leading to blindness
Pain	Headache	Retro-orbital
Blind spot	Enlarged	Central scotoma
Pupils	Normal	Afferent pupillary defect

Visual Field Defects

Be confident of detecting the common field defects in clinical practice:

- Homonymous hemianopia
- Bitemporal hemianopia
- Upper and lower quadrantic hemianopia
- Scotoma.

Even when there is only perception of light, visual field defects must be looked for. Use a 5 mm white hat pin to determine the visual fields and a red pin for scotoma. A good indication of the presence of a visual field defect can be quickly noted by the candidate by comparing their visual field with the patients with both eyes open – confrontation, using only finger movements.

By using simultaneous finger movements in the upper quadrants of both sides and then the lower quadrants, the candidate will be able to detect:

- Gross upper and lower quadrantic hemianopia
- Homonymous hemianopia
- Bitemporal hemianopia
- Visual inattention.

Central Scotoma

Common causes are:

- Optic neuritis, retrobulbar neuritis, often without other features of multiple sclerosis
- Optic atrophy.

Optic Atrophy

This may be due to:

- **Optic Nerve Compression:**
    - Olfactory groove meningioma
    - Sphenoidal ridge meningioma
    - Optic nerve glioma
- **Toxins:**
    - Tobacco
    - Methyl alcohol
- **Vitamin Deficiencies:**
    - Vitamin B1
    - Vitamin B12
- **Congenital:** Leber's hereditary optic atrophy
- **Trauma**
- **Ischaemia:**
    - central retinal artery occlusion
    - ischaemic optic neuropathy
- **Neurosyphilis**

Junctional Scotoma

A junctional scotoma is produced by lesions of the anterior chiasma compressing:

- The papillo-macular bundle producing an ipsilateral scotoma

- The forward looping lower nasal fibres, producing a contralateral upper temporal defect (see Fig 47).

It is important to look for a contralateral upper quadrantic defect in all patients with unilateral blindness, central scotoma or unilateral primary optic atrophy and consider the possibility of a compressive lesion of the anterior chiasma.

Concentric Diminution of the Field of Vision

When severe it will produce **'tunnel vision' or 'tubular vision'.** It is common in non-organic blindness but may also be seen in:

- Papilloedema
- Glaucoma
- Retinal disease – choroidoretinitis, retinitis pigmentosa.

Quadrantic Field Defects

This is due to involvement of fibres sweeping from the lateral geniculate body to the visual cortex. The upper fibres sweep through the parietal lobe and lower fibres through the temporal lobe. The defect is congruous.

Temporal lobe lesions → upper quadrantic hemianopia
Parietal lobe lesions → lower quadrantic hemianopia.

See Fig 48.

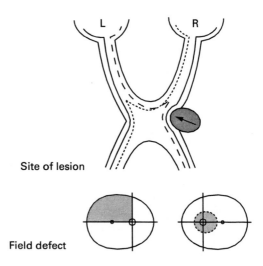

Figure 47: Junctional scotoma – site of lesion and field defect

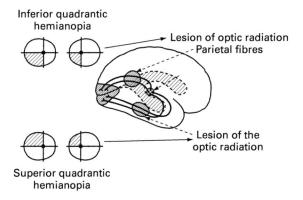

Inferior quadrantic
hemianopia

Lesion of optic radiation
Parietal fibres

Lesion of the
optic radiation

Superior quadrantic
hemianopia

Figure 48: Quadrantic field defects

Homonymous Hemianopia

The patient does not see one half of the visual field – left or right. In the left homonymous hemianopia the patient does not see the left half of the visual field.

This is apparent when the visual field of the left eye is tested, the right eye is tested or the visual field is tested with both eyes open. (This is of greater clinical significance than saying there is a temporal defect in the left eye and a nasal defect in the right eye.)

The lesion producing an homonymous hemianopia is either in the optic tract or radiation.

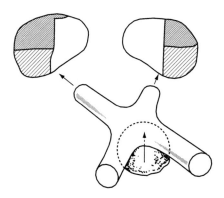

Figure 49: Bitemporal hemianopia due to pituitary tumour

- Optic tract → incongruous hemianopia
- Optic radiation → congruous hemianopia
- Optic tract lesions may be produced by pituitary tumour, craniopharyngioma, chordoma and meningioma
- Optic radiation lesions are usually due to a tumour or infarction in the middle cerebral territory
- Visual cortex lesions produce a macular sparing homonymous hemianopia and may occur with migraine and posterior cerebral ischaemia

Temporal Hemianopia

A temporal hemianopia may be unilateral or bilateral and is due to chiasmatic compression. The latter is the more commonly recognised clinical abnormality.

When there is compression from above (craniopharyngioma) the lower fields are affected first and more.

When there is compression from below (the pituitary tumour) the upper fields are affected first and the lower fields later – see Fig. 49.

Sudden Blindness

Ocular Causes

- Trauma
- Acute glaucoma
- Retinal detachment
- Vitreous haemorrhage (diabetes)

Neuro-ophthalmic Causes

- Toxins – methyl alcohol
- Vascular – retinal artery thrombosis or embolism, cranial arteritis, central retinal vein thrombosis
- Optic neuritis and retrobulbar neuritis
- Acute optic nerve compression

Visual Defect by Site of Lesion

SITE	DEFICIT
Retina	Scotoma
Macula	'Blindness' (PL, NPL)
Optic nerve	Scotoma
	Altitudinal defect
	Afferent pupillary defect
Optic chiasma	Temporal hemianopia
	Junctional scotoma
Optic tract	Incongruous hemianopia
Optic radiation	Congruous hemianopia
Occipital lobe	Congruous hemianopia with macular sparing, hemianopic scotoma

Non-organic Blindness

This may be present with the following.

Unilateral Blindness

The patient claims that they do not see the ipsilateral half of the visual field with both eyes open – as in a true homonymous hemianopia. When the visual fields are tested, they claim there is no vision when only the affected eye is open.

(Lay individuals and some in the medical profession are under the impression that each eye contributes to the corresponding half of the visual field.)

Total Bilateral Blindness

The person pretends not to see at all and bumps into objects wilfully. The menace reflex and pupillary reflex are retained, while the optic fundi and visual evoked responses are normal.

Tunnel Vision

In tunnel vision due to non-organic causes, the intact vision is a clear-cut tube – the diameter of retained vision is the same at all distances. In organic tunnel vision, it is more in the form of a cone from the eye, with retained vision increasing with distance (see Fig 50).

HISTORY TAKING STATION

Any of the conditions just mentioned may be present.

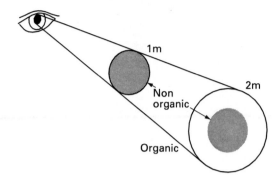

Figure 50: Tunnel vision

Determine the Exact Defect of Vision

The Visual Impairment in Daily Life

Blurred vision: Too non-specific to be of diagnostic or localising value

Confined to one eye: Has the patient closed each eye in turn to note the vision in the unaffected eye and to ascertain that it is a defect in one eye and not a defect in one half of the field of vision?

Visual field defect: This is best seen by asking the patient for the defect noted with both eyes open. If it is:

- **Homonymous hemianopia,** the patient is unable to see objects to the left or right of the mid line. If there is macular involvement, the object in the field of central vision is split.
- **Lower quadrantic hemianopia,** the patient does not see objects in the lower half of the visual field and may kick them
- **Upper quadrantic hemianopia,** the patient does not see objects in the upper quadrant of field of vision
- **Bitemporal hemianopia,** the patient does not see the objects in the periphery on both sides
- **Tunnel or tubular vision,** this is similar to bitemporal hemianopia but is more restricted.

'Black spots': Spots or patches of impaired vision are due to scotoma. This may be central in the central scotoma.

	Normal	Primary optic atrophy	Optic neuritis	Papilloerdema	Secondary optic atrophy
Contour	well demarcated	very clear cut	blurred	blurred	ill defined
Colour	pinkish	white	very pink	very pink	pale
Optic cup	seen well	not seen	not seen	not seen	not seen
Circulation	V:A = 3:2	narrow arteries	normal	veins dilated	veins dilated
Curiosities	normal macula	normal macula		haemorrhages	haemorrhages
Vision	normal VA, VF Normal blind spot Normal colour vis	blind, scotoma impaired VA	blind scotoma impaired VA	may be normal enlarged B spot impaired colour Tubular vision	blind, scotoma impaired VA

OPTIC FUNDI

Duration and Onset

The duration given by the patient may be inaccurate if it is an incidental discovery by them or the medical attendant. It is important to find out the exact situation when the deficit was first discovered.

Progress

It is extremely important to know whether vision is getting better or worse – ask for objective evidence as to why the patient feels it is getting better or worse.

Correction by Refraction

Find out whether the vision is improved with glasses and whether there has been an optical consultation and if so, what were the results?

Associated Symptoms

- Pain
- Headache
- Double vision
- Ptosis
- Other neurological symptoms

Plan of Action

What has been suggested to the patient and what do you think should be the plan of action – which depends to a large extent on the nature of the defect.

DISORDERS OF HEARING

NEUROLOGY STATION

First determine whether hearing is faulty by testing with the:

- Whispered voice – in each ear
- Ticking of a wrist watch.

Once you have established there is impaired hearing, find out whether it is:

- Nerve deafness
- Conductive or middle ear deafness.

Use a tuning fork (256 or 512, not the 128 Hz used for vibration sense), and carry out the following two tests.

Weber's Test

This tests hearing by conduction through the bone only – it is not interfered by disease of the middle ear or ossicles.

The tuning fork is kept on the vertex or middle of the forehead. If hearing is normal it is heard equally in both ears. If heard better in the normal ear there is nerve deafness in the other. If heard better in the deaf ear there is conductive deafness in that ear.

Rinne's Test

A 512 or 1024 Hz tuning fork is held on the mastoid until it is no longer heard and then close to the external auditory meatus, when it will be heard by the normal individual, as air conduction is better than bone conduction.

This could also be verified by asking the patient whether the sound is better heard with the fork on the mastoid or in front of the ear. In conductive or middle ear deafness, the tuning fork is heard better over the mastoid.

If air conduction is better than bone conduction (AC>BC) this means that there is nerve deafness (AC>BC in normal individuals as well).

If bone conduction is better than air conduction (BC>AC), this means that there is conductive or middle ear deafness.

HISTORY TAKING STATION

Patients with disease of the VIII nerve (tinnitus, deafness, vertigo) must be examined carefully for evidence of cerebello-pontine angle signs with raised intracranial pressure. Look for:

- Papilloedema
- Ophthalmic sensory loss including corneal reflex
- Ipsilateral VI,VII palsy
- Ipsilateral cerebellar signs
- Bilateral pyramidal signs.

From the history it may be possible to determine whether the deafness is conductive or sensory-neural and occasionally the cause.

It is important to find out how it was first detected and whether:

- Hearing in each ear was checked by the patient
- Others had noted deafness
- There is differential hearing loss for particular sounds
- Sound is heard well but speech discrimination is poor
- It is unilateral or bilateral
- A hearing aid has helped.

Accompanying symptoms

Accompanying symptoms may help to determine the site and cause of the disorder.

For the site

- **Middle ear:** Earache, ear discharge
- **Inner ear:** Tinnitus, ability to hear some sounds, not others (whispered voice heard but not high frequency sounds like the ticking of a watch), loudness recruitment – the difference between the affected and unaffected ear is more obvious with soft sounds rather than with loud sounds, vertigo.
- **Auditory nerve:** Tinnitus, hyperacusis if the facial nerve is affected in the facial canal before supply to the stapedius muscle, and loss of taste in anterior two thirds of the tongue if the chorda tympani branch of facial nerve is affected.
- **Cerebellopontine angle:** Tinnitus, vertigo, ataxia, headache if there is raised intracranial pressure

For the causes

- **Temporal profile:** Whether acute, fluctuating or slowly progressive. Episodic vertigo with vomiting and progressive deafness occurs with Ménière's disease.
- **Family history of deafness**
- **History of trauma with bleeding from ear**
- **Vesicles of herpes in external auditory meatus and fauces**
- **Drug history:** Particularly antibiotics like neomycin and aminoglycosides

VERTIGO

NEUROLOGY STATION

Sites of Lesion

- External ear
- Middle ear
- Labyrinth
- Vestibular nerve
  - internal ear
  - posterior fossa
- Brain stem
- Temporal lobe

(See also nystagmus and bulbar palsy, on pages 113 and 130.)

Vertigo is an hallucination of motion, usually experienced as a sensation of rotation and occasionally as rolling, rocking, swaying, or a movement inside the head. Whether the sensation is one of subject rotating (subjective vertigo) or surrounding objects moving is not of clinical significance.

Vertigo is produced by disorders of the labyrinth, vestibular nerve or its central connections in the brain stem and temporal lobes. Vertigo commonly occurs with acute disorders at these sites and may be absent or mild in chronic disorders.

Common causes are:

- **Benign paroxysmal vertigo:** Vertigo may be brief and positional, without cochlear (tinnitus, deafness) or cerebello-pontine angle symptoms or signs.
- **Acute labyrinthitis:** Vertigo may be accompanied by tinnitus. An ear infection may be the cause.
- **Vestibular neuronitis:** This is vertigo without cochlear manifestations.
- **Cerebello-pontine angle lesions:** Vertigo is late and mild unless the lesion is acute. CP angle signs will predominate.
- **Brain stem lesions:** This occurs particularly in lateral medullary syndrome secondary to ischaemia where there is associated vomiting, dysarthria, dysphagia and nasal regurgitation.

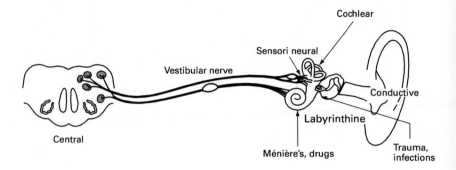

Figure 51: Vertigo

Examination of Vertiginous Patient

External Ear Including External Auditory Meatus
- Vesicles
- Evidence of inflammation
- Wax
- Tenderness over tragus
- Discharge

Tympanic Membrane
- Rupture
- Inflammation

Internal Ear and VIII Nerve
- Deafness
- Rinne's test
- Weber's test

Cerebello-pontine Angle
- Cerebellar signs
- Pontine and pontine angle signs:
  - Ophthalmic V
    - sensory impairment
    - corneal reflex
  - VI nerve
  - VII nerve
  - Pyramidal signs

Raised Intracranial Pressure

- Papilloedema

HISTORY TAKING STATION

The history is directed towards determining the site of the lesion and the disease process.

Confirm Vertigo

The usual symptom is giddiness, dizziness or an equivalent term. Confirm that there is a sensation of motion, which is not necessarily rotational. Whether it is 'subjective' (perceived motion is of 'patient') or objective (motion is of 'environment') is not of diagnostic significance.

Duration

This is not of differential significance.

Associated Symptoms

These are very significant. Specific complaints to be asked about include:

- Tinnitus
- Deafness
- Numbness of face
- Diplopia
- Ataxia and inco-ordination
- Vesicles in and around the ear
- Headache and vomiting.

Past History

- Vertigo
- Any of the above associated symptoms
- Recurrence of attacks with profuse vomiting and prostration with a background of tinnitus and progressive deafness

SENSORY
DISTURBANCES

SITES AND DISTURBANCES

NEUROLOGY STATION

Sensory disturbances are less common than motor disturbances, particularly in an examination setting. They are more difficult to evaluate, as sensory signs are subject dependent and need the co-operation of the patient.

Disorders which are primarily in the muscle (myopathies) and the AHC (disease of the motor neurone) are usually devoid of sensory signs. Neurologically speaking an 'ache', unless well localised, is not of localising significance. Skin lesions may be accompanied by sensory symptoms and sensory signs which do not conform to a nerve or dermatomal pattern.

Myopathies

Muscular dystrophies are devoid of sensory symptoms and signs but inflammatory myopathies may have localised muscle pain and tenderness with other features of inflammation. Metabolic myopathies could have muscle pain.

Myasthenia

This is devoid of sensory symptoms and signs.

Neuropathies

Symptom: There is numbness rather than pain. It is distal in peripheral neuropathies and localised in mononeuropathies.

Signs: There is a 'glove and stocking' sensory impairment with impaired vibration and position sense in peripheral neuropathies. It is localised to the distribution of the nerve in mononeuropathies.

NERVE	DISTRIBUTION
Ulnar nerve	Little finger, ulnar 1/2 of ring finger, ulnar aspect of hand.
Median nerve	Lateral aspect of palm, thumb, index and middle fingers on palmar surface, distal phalanx of same fingers on dorsal side.
Radial nerve	First dorsal interosseous space.
Common peroneal	Dorsum of foot and outer leg.
Sural nerve	Outer heel.

Carpal Tunnel Syndrome

This is the most common cause of numbness of the hand and the most common neurological complication of pregnancy. As the history is 'classical' it could be given in the history taking station.

Symptom: Often it is a middle aged obese lady who complains of numbness of one or both hands, particularly at night and with any activity which requires a closed fist like writing, gripping, wringing clothes, etc. The numbness often affects all fingers and is not confined to the fingers supplied by the median nerve, though it is due to compression of the median nerve.

Signs: There may be impairment of sensation in median nerve distribution or all the fingers. Wasting is late and is seen in about 1% of patients. It is confined to the outer aspect of the thenar eminence.

Confirmation: This is by electrophysiology. Sensory nerve conduction is reduced and there is an increased latency of median nerve conduction at the wrist – normal is up to about 4 mSec.

Meralgia Paraesthetica

This is the second most common neurological complication of pregnancy. It is due to compression of the lateral cutaneous nerve of the thigh at the inguinal ligament usually accompanying the lordosis of pregnancy or disc prolapse.

Symptom: There is a burning sensation in a longitudinal oval area on the outer aspect of the thigh.

Signs: There is a sensory impairment in the same area accompanied by lordosis.

Radiculopathies

There is pain, sometimes excruciating, in root distribution. The radiation is accurately localised with lumbar and thoracic radiculopathies but less well localised in cervical radiculopathy (see Figs 52 and 53 for dermatomal patterns).

Root pains bilaterally at the same level produce a constricting band-like sensation – 'girdle pains'. These are usually indicative of a compressive lesion, pressing on the dorsal nerve roots.

Bilateral sciatica has the same significance as girdle pains and are seen most often with a central disc prolapse compressing the nerve roots bilaterally.

Some polyradiculopathies, notably tuberculous polyradiculopathy associated with marked cerebrospinal fluid (CSF) protein elevation may present with intolerable paraesthesiae and hyperaesthesiae.

Root pains are often aggravated by manoeuvres which increase intraspinal pressure like:

L aughing
S neezing
C oughing
S training

– remember as LSCS (the same as in Lower Segment Caesarian Section).

Sign-Sensory Impairment in Dermatome Distribution

NERVE ROOT	DISTRIBUTION
C5	Outer upper arm
C6	Outer forearm, thumb, index finger
C7	Middle finger
C8,T1	Little finger, ulnar 1/2 of ring finger, ulnar aspect of palm, ulnar forearm to elbow
L1	Groin and upper thigh
L2	Upper thigh anteriorly
L3	Mid thigh anteriorly
L4	Across knee, medial lower leg
L5	Lateral lower leg, dorsum of foot
S1	Sole of foot and little toe
S2,3,4	Saddle area

Spinal Cord Lesions

Brown Sequard

There is hemichord affection with ipsilateral loss of position and vibration sense with contralateral loss of pain and temperature.

With Sensory Level

The sensory level is the level below which all modalities of sensation are impaired or lost. It may be preceded by features of Brown Séquard syndrome or a hypaesthetic level, which may persist. A sensory level is often seen in the thorax or abdomen in the thoracic cord compression or in upper limbs in the cervical (see Fig 3 on page 11).

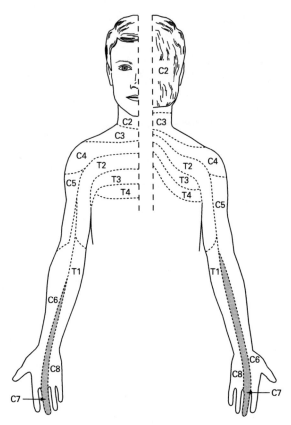

Figure 52: UL dermatomes

Dissociate Sensory Loss

This is a suspended sensory loss with dissociation of modalities of sensation lost – usually pain and temperature loss with preserved touch, vibration and position sense.

It is classically seen in syringomyelia with spino-thalamic tract involvement with preserved posterior columns. It can occur with intramedullary lesions anywhere in the spinal cord. It also occurs in the brain stem up to the pontine level where the posterior column fibres and spinothalamic fibres unite to form the single medial leminiscus (see Fig 30 on page 71).

Saddle Sensory Loss

This occurs in cauda equina lesions with associated S2, S3 and S4 motor and sphincter signs (see Fig 6 on page 18).

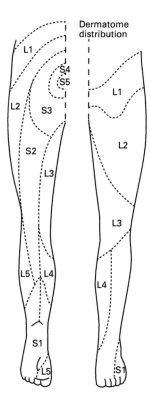

Figure 53: Sensation (modified from Aids to the Examination of the Peripheral Nervous System)

It needs to be differentiated from sacral sensory loss of extradural compression at higher levels with other localising signs.

Posterior Column Loss Only

This occurs with tabes dorsalis and subacute combined degeneration of the cord, presenting with sensory ataxia and Rombergism. The 'wash basin sign' is the equivalent symptom and accompanies a positive Romberg's sign.

Brain Stem Lesions

Pons and Medulla

These produce an ipsilateral facial pain with impairment of pain sensation 'anesthesia dolorosa'. This is accompanied by loss of pain sensation on the opposite side of the body – 'checker board type of anaesthesia'.

163

Mid Brain

There is numbness, coldness or warmth of the contralateral face, arm and legs with reduced pain and temperature of the face, arm and leg.

Thalamus

Symptom: A deep pain diffusely on the opposite side of the body.

Signs: In hyperpathia pain threshold is raised but when it is exceeded there is an unpleasant quality. There is also impaired pain, temperature and touch sensation. Choreo-athetosis and a homonymous hemianopia may accompany it.

Internal Capsule

Symptom: There is a contralateral sensory disturbance of the face, arm and leg.

Signs: Look for impaired pain, temperature and touch with associated hemiplegia and homonymous hemianopia.

Sensory Cortex

Symptom: Numbness is localised to a limb or part of a limb and there is a sensory Jacksonian epilepsy.

Signs: There is an impaired localisation of touch, two point discrimination, stereognosis, and position sense.

Parietal Lobe

Parietal lobe lesions do not produce crude sensory symptoms related to pain, temperature and touch. There is difficulty in localising and identifying objects without visual help (e.g. in the dark, coins in the pocket, etc).

There is also a lack of spatial orientation and apraxia for purposive movements like dressing.

Signs

Look for loss of:

- One point discrimination – identifying texture
- Two point discrimination – 1cm on fingers, 3 cm on soles of shodden feet

- Three point discrimination – stereognosis
- Accurate localisation of touch.

HISTORY TAKING STATION

Please read the neurology station on sensory disturbances for causes and differential features (see page 159).

In the history of a patient with sensory complaints, ask specifically for the following.

Nature of the Sensory Complaint

Is it a:

- Pain?
- Numbness and tingling?
- Burning or unpleasant ache?
- Loss of feeling or touch and pain sensation – any painless burns?
- Inability to appreciate warmth or cold?
- Hypersensitive or unpleasant quality?
- Radiation of pain?
- Present at rest or
- Made better or worse by standing, walking, climbing and cycling?

Localisation

Is the above complaint:

- Over a localised area; and if so
- Is it in the distribution of a particular nerve; or
- Particular nerve root or roots – e.g. over thigh or 'saddle area'
- Is it distal involving feet and hands – 'glove and stocking'
- Affecting the entire arm – 'coat sleeve'
- Below a certain level
- A bizarre or patchy distribution
- Neuralgic – sharp, shooting, stabbing or 'lightning pains'
- Preceded or accompanied by a skin lesion?

Aggravating and Relieving Factors

Is the pain aggravated by:

- Laughing, straining, coughing, sneezing – if in root distribution?

Is the pain relieved by:

- Ordinary analgesics?
- Anti-depressants?
- Carbamazepine?

SCIATICA AND LUMBAR DISC PROLAPSE

NEUROLOGY STATION

Sciatica is a well delineated radiating root pain, usually in the distribution of the L5 or S1 nerve root. The radiation of the pain is often well localised by the patient, as shown below:

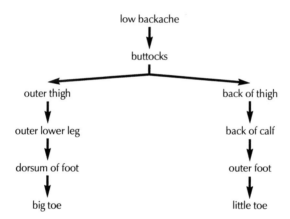

ROOT PAIN
5th Lumbar (L5)   1st Sacral (S1)

low backache
↓
buttocks

outer thigh   back of thigh
↓   ↓
outer lower leg   back of calf
↓   ↓
dorsum of foot   outer foot
↓   ↓
big toe   little toe

There are **accompanying** signs, again depending on the root of affection.

Signs

L5	S1
Foot drop	Claw foot
Dorsiflexors weak	Plantar flexors weak
Wasting of tibialis anterior ±	Calf wasting ±
KJ, AJ normal	AJ impaired/absent
Plantar normal	Impaired or absent
Sensory impairment	Sensory impairment
Dorsum of foot	Sole of foot

Levels of Root Lesions

Spinal Canal

L5 and S1 arise from the spinal cord opposite T12 and L1 vertebrae. So there is a long course inside the spinal canal from T12 to S1.

In the lesions opposite T12 and L1, both the spinal cord and roots (high cauda equina lesion) will be involved and only the roots in lesions lower than L1 – low cauda equina lesions.

The high cauda equina lesions will have both LMN and UMN signs. The lesion may be due to a tumour or lumbar disc prolapse. Posterolateral disc protrusion will result in unilateral root compression, while central disc protrusion may compress roots bilaterally.

Pelvis

Space-occupying lesions of the pelvic organs could press the root/s, the sacral plexus or sciatic nerve.

Sciatic Nerve

This may be damaged in the buttocks by a wrongly located intramuscular injection into the buttock or in the thigh by a neurofibroma.

Peripheral Nerve

L5 may be involved in the common peroneal and S1 in the posterior tibial nerve lesions.

Lumbar Disc Prolapse

The most common lumbar discs to prolapse are L4/L5 and L5/S1. The prolapse may be central or more often posterolateral compressing roots unilaterally.

An L4/L5 disc usually compresses the L5 nerve root and an L5/S1 disc compresses the S1 nerve root. An L4/L5 disc can compress both L5 and S1 nerve roots but an L5/S1 cannot compress the L5 nerve root which is at a higher level.

Note that the common lumbar disc prolapse cannot compress the spinal cord which ends at L1 level, so this is not a cause of paraparesis.

Symptoms

Common presenting symptoms include the following.

- Low backache
- Sciatica – radiation of pain depends on the nerve root compressed
- Meralgia paraesthetica
- Occasionally foot drop or weakness of plantar flexion
- Neurogenic intermittent claudication
- Bladder and sexual dysfunction, but this is extremely uncommon

Signs

See under sciatica – L5 or S1 root signs, on page 167.

Claudication – Ischaemic vs Neurogenic

	ISCHAEMIC	NEUROGENIC
Main symptom	Pain	Numbness
Site	Localised	Radiates
"	Foot, calf, thigh	Foot → buttock or
"	Buttock	buttock → foot
At rest	Symptoms ±	Symptoms absent
Standing	Symptom same	Often appear
Walking	Symptom worse	Symptom worse
Cycling	Worse	Better
Pulses	Diminished	Normal
CNS signs	Absent	May be present
Stretch signs	Absent	± at rest
Motor signs	Absent	± after walking
Sensory signs	Absent	± after walking
Ankle jerk	Normal	± after walking
Cause	Arterial stenosis or occlusion	Lumbar canal stenosis or cauda equina tumour

Investigations for Disc Prolapse

- **Plain films:** May show a narrowing of L4/5 or L5/S1 disc space. There may be associated spondylolisthesis or reverse spondylolisthesis.
- **Myelography:** Now used only when Magnetic Resonance Imaging (MRI) facilities are not available.
- **CT scans and CT myelography:** Used only when MRI is not available. Only axial pictures are obtained.
- **MRI scanning:** The investigation of choice. It has the advantage of showing the films in the longitudinal axis from the cervical to sacral region as well as showing transverse slices. It does not require lumbar puncture and radio-opaque dyes.

Deciding on the Need for Disc Surgery

Not all patients with sciatica need surgery. Those who may require surgical treatment include the following:

- Failed medical treatment which may include adequate rest in bed, traction, a lumbosacral support and analgesics
- Bilateral sciatica indicative of a large central disc prolapse
- Neurogenic intermittent claudication
- When physical signs are indicative of objective evidence of root compression
- Patient demand: A young active patient may refuse prolonged conservative management which restricts activities.

A positive stretch test (straight leg raising test) in itself is not indicative of the need for surgery, though it may give some indication of the severity of the sciatica.

HISTORY TAKING STATION

Please read the neurology station on sciatica (page 167) for sites of lesions, causes and differential features.

The following interrogation will help to determine the nerve root involved, the level and the probable cause.

- How was the pain precipitated – bending, lifting a heavy object?
- Does it conform to the L5 distribution or S1?
- Is it present at rest?
- What happens on standing, walking, climbing stairs and cycling?
- Has there been curvature of the spine – scoliosis?
- Is there ascending or descending numbness of the legs on standing for some time or walking?
- What is the severity of the pain? The degree can be assessed by the amount of interference with work and activities of daily living (ADL).
- What investigations were carried out?
- What is the plan of management as advised by the attending physician?
- Has there been a surgical opinion?

GENERAL

EXAMINATION TO EXCLUDE A SIGNIFICANT INTRACRANIAL LESION IN A PATIENT WITH COMMON GENERAL SYMPTOMS

Such symptoms include a headache, attacks of loss of consciousness and falls.

A head to toe detailed neurological examination does not always seem necessary in patients showing general symptoms like headache, episodes of loss of consciousness and falls.

The following facets of examination are important to exclude raised intracranial pressure and a structural focal lesion.

The majority of patients presenting with such symptoms may not have abnormal physical signs, nevertheless they could be given at the PACES examination. This is to assess whether the candidate is able to do a meaningful and relevant, clinical examination rather than a detailed routine CNS examination.

Such an examination should include:

- **Gait:** A unilateral abnormality in gait as in hemiparesis
- **Funduscopic examination:** For papilloedema, optic atrophy
- **Visual fields:** Using the confrontation method would be adequate to detect the upper and lower quadrantic hemianopia, homonymous hemianopia and bitemporal hemianopia, which are important clinical defects
- **Facial palsy :** Usually the UMN type
- **Outstretched hands:** For drift, hypotonia, tremors, followed by the finger nose test
- **Finger nose test:** For cerebellar signs
- **Power:** Weakness of the hand as determined by grip and shoulders (abduction)

- **Legs**: Weakness of the proximal muscles as noted in getting up from a chair or squat, weakness of distal muscles as noted on walking on toes or heels
- **Reflexes**: Supinator jerk and knee jerk, and plantars are of particular importance.

HISTORY TAKING STATION – HEADACHE

The diagnosis depends on a good history and the following facets need to be questioned. Initially 'let the patient speak' and if some of the questions below are not answered the candidate could ask direct questions.

Duration

- **Total duration:** How long has the patient had the headaches – days, weeks, months or years?
- **Duration of each episode:** How long has each episode lasted?

Onset

It is particularly important to find out whether the onset of the headache was acute and whether the patient can 'time it to the minute', as happens in vascular headaches, especially SAH.

Severity

How severe is the headache? Assess this by asking the patient if they need to rest, sleep or keep away from work.

Nature

- Is the headache continued or intermittent?
- Is there an ache, pain or throbbing?

Frequency

How many times does the headache occur per day, week or month?

Time of Day

It is important to find out whether it is an awakening or a nocturnal headache disturbing sleep – this suggests raised intracranial pressure.

Site of Headache

Is it diffuse or more localised? Common sites are frontal, bitemporal, unilateral, vertical, occipito-cervical and band-like.

Associated Symptoms

Vomiting is of particular importance (headache, vomiting and papilloedema is the triad for raised intracranial pressure). It is also important to find out whether there are any focal neurological symptoms like abnormalities of speech, vision, motor and sensory symptoms.

Aggravating Factors

Activities which raise intracranial pressure are laughing, straining, coughing, sneezing (LSCS) and would aggravate a headache associated with raised intracranial pressure.

Relieving Factors

What does the patient do to relieve the headache?

Family History

A family history of headache may be present with migraine. It is not uncommon for family members, particularly children, to develop headaches when a family member or close friend has had a serious intracranial illness with headaches.

The above features may be remembered in one sentence as TONS FDAAF:

T ime
O nset
N ature
S ite
F requency
D uration
A ccompanying and
A ggravating
F actors

are of importance.

HISTORY TAKING STATION – LOSS OF CONSCIOUSNESS

As this is a common problem, it is easy to find patients with this presentation for the history taking station and the neurology clinical station.

The relevant examination needed is as given on page 173. As for headaches, the examination may not reveal any positive signs and the diagnosis is very much dependent on a good history.

While with a headache patient the axiom is to 'let the patient speak', in presentations with loss of consciousness a reliable eye witness account directly from the witness or indirectly from the patient is of utmost value.

The history is directed at differentiating a seizure from other common paroxysmal conditions:

- Fits
- Faints
- Pseudoseizures
- Drop attacks
- Funny turns
- Other paroxysmal conditions
- Cause in doubt.

Unless the history is taken in detail, the cause will be in doubt in many instances as neither the examination nor investigations will reveal an abnormality.

There are three stages for which a detailed history is necessary:

- Aura or premonitory phase
- The episode or ictus
- Post ictal phase – 'after the attack'.

Premonitory Phase or 'Aura' and Bio-data

Let us consider each phase in detail.

	FIT	PSEUDO FIT	FAINT
Age	Any age	Commonly young female	Uncommon in young males
Family history	May be present	Of true fit +/–	Usually not
Duration	None or short	May be long	May be adequate to avoid a fall
Location	Anywhere, could be in dangerous location	Always in company	Closed, humid room Bad locations avoided
In sleep	May occur	Never	Never
Posture	May occur when seated or lying	Any position	Usually standing
Provocative	Sleep deprivation	Lack of attention	Hunger and fatigue

The 'Ictus' or Event

	FIT	PSEUDO FIT	FAINT
Colour	Normal or flushed	Normal	Pale
Sweating	0	0	+/–
Tone	Tonic or clonic	Stiff, aggressive	Flaccid
Head and eyes	May be deviated	Deviated or tightly closed	Blank, staring
Duration	5–30 minutes	May be long	Usually less than 5 minutes
Injuries	Mucosal – tongue, Lips, head	Superficial +/–	Usually absent or superficial
Frothing	+/–	+/–	0
Incontinence	+/–	+/–	Usually absent

Post-ictal Phase

	FIT	PSEUDO FIT	FAINT
Duration	>30 minutes	Variable	Few minutes
Activity	Drowsy or sleeps	Demanding Aggression +/–	Near normal
Headache	+/–	May pretend	0
Amnesia	+	May pretend	0
Automatism	Rarely	+/–	0

Pathognomonic features of a true seizure which distinguishes it from a faint or pseudo-seizure include occurrence:

- In sleep
- While alone
- In unsavoury or dangerous locations – at heights, on the road, near fire, etc
- Mucosal or serious injuries.

Note: A person, medically qualified or one who has carefully observed a seizure, can use saliva to froth and voluntarily pass urine to give the impression that there has been incontinence. So frothing and incontinence does not confirm that an ictus is a true seizure. While it is possible for an experienced clinician to detect a pseudo-seizure when they see one, it may be difficult to be certain on an eye witness account.

HISTORY TAKING STATION – FALLS

The causes of falls vary with age – falls in childhood have totally different causes to those in the elderly, while they are uncommon in healthy adults.

Falls are due to one of the following reasons:

- Weakness of lower limbs
- Instability at joints
- Involuntary movements
- Seizure activity
- Unsteadiness
- Vertigo
- Loss of postural tone without loss of consciousness
- Postural hypotension
- Unsteadiness
- Environmental factors – slipping, pushed or pulled.

Before determining the probable cause of the fall, it is advantageous to find out which one of the above points was responsible for the fall.

Except in situations where there has been loss of consciousness or retrograde amnesia, the patient will be able to describe the event in detail if properly questioned.

A reliable eye witness account will be useful especially where recall is poor.

Questions should be asked in a chronological manner so that the event is replayed. Obtain adequate details – the following questions are helpful.

What Were You Doing When You Fell?

This question will reveal:

- Location
- Posture at time of falling
- Activity just before the fall
- Premonitory symptoms, if any, before the fall
- Did the patient warn bystanders/witnesses?

What Do You Recall of the Falling Process?

Those who fall due to loss of consciousness or seizure activity will not recall the falling process.

How Long Were You on the Ground?

All except those who were unconscious will be able to tell the time spent on the ground.

How Did You Get Up?

Most except those who have had a 'drop attack' or transient disturbance other than a seizure, will need some form of assistance to get up.

Then What Happened or How Did You Feel After You Got Up?

The following are useful to tell the difference between each cause:

- Able to resume activity
- Confused or amnesic
- Drowsy or sleepy
- Headache
- Pale and sweaty
- Vomiting
- Weakness of limbs continued to a greater, lesser or same extent
- Need for hospitalisation, investigation and treatment with sedation or IV fluids.

Did You Have Any Falls Before? If So, What Were the Circumstances?

This should consolidate the information obtained of the last fall which the patient should be able to recall vividly.

Falls in Children

- **'Accidents' during play:** This is the most common cause but it is not of medical significance
- **Faints:** This is the next most common fall. It usually happens while standing for long periods without breakfast
- **Hypoglycaemia:** Probably not as common as suspected
- **Seizures:** Includes myoclonic varieties. There are some 'seizures' which tend to occur with contact or minimal trauma
- **Myopathies:** This may be the presentation of Duchenne's dystrophy
- **SSPE (subacute sclerosing panencephalitis):** This may be the presenting feature before myoclonic jerks become obvious
- **Vertigo:** This is an uncommon cause

Falls in the Elderly

This is not an uncommon symptom late in life. The common causes are:

- Vertigo
- Difficulty in changing posture from the standing to sitting posture or sitting to standing position, due to a weakness of proximal muscles. There is no loss of consciousness. The person may need assistance to get up.

Ataxia

- Difficulty in propulsion – Parkinson's disease
- Drop attacks – the person 'drops' to the ground without warning but is able to get up almost immediately, though there is a momentary loss of consciousness and amnesia for the falling process. It is usually seen in vertebro-basilar ischaemia which may be precipitated by the head turning in cervical spondylotics. It may also occur with Parkinson's disease.
- Postural hypotension – particularly with those on anti-hypertensives
- Hypoglycaemia – particularly with diabetics on treatment
- Syncope – including carotid sinus syncope
- Late onset seizures

Examination in a Patient with Falls

A patient with falls could be given either at the cardiovascular or the neurological systems. Both systems need careful examination.

Complete examination of the **cardiovascular system** including:

- Listening for bruits over the carotids and the vertebrals. The latter is auscultated over the supra-clavicular fossae.

- Detection of subclavian steal syndrome by palpating both radial pulses and checking blood pressure in both arms
- Examining for arrhythmias
- Postural hypotension.

Specific facets of the nervous system, needing special attention are:

- Observing patient sitting and standing
- Difficulties in initiating walking and shuffling and other features of Parkinson's disease
- Tandem ataxia
- Tremors at rest and also on volition, as in the finger nose test
- Gower's sign
- Cerebello-pontine angle signs – see page 154
- Examination as for other general symptoms – see page 173.

NEUROLOGY STATION – DEMENTIA

When confronted with a patient with poor memory and deteriorating intellect, it is important to determine:

- Whether there is in fact an impairment of higher function and memory?
- If present, how severe is it? Try to quantify it. Is it progressive or deteriorating?
- Is there a treatable cause?

(The Folstein mini mental scale is useful for both the first and second bullet points.)

Do not be satisfied with a diagnosis of senile dementia until all treatable causes are excluded, particularly in those who are not 'senile.' Dementia should be considered a symptom rather than a diagnosis, and should be investigated fully.

It is useful to test the following and quantify (using a modified Folstein mini mental scale).

Orientation in Time

- Approximate time
- Date
- Day
- Month
- Year

(One point each – total five points)

Orientation in Space and Person

- Name of ward or clinic
- Name of hospital
- Place/city
- Country
- Name of doctor

(One point each – total five points)

Short Term Memory

Show three objects and ask the patient to name them, after removing them from view. (One point each – total three points.)

Attention and Calculation

Subtract 7 from 100 serially. Give one point for each correct answer. Stop after five answers (five points).

Recall

Ask for the names of the three objects shown earlier after about five minutes (three points).

Language and Speech

- **Naming:** Two common objects. One point each (two points).
- **Obeying a 3-stage verbal command:** For example, ask the patient 'with your finger, touch your nose and then the ear'. Do not specify the finger or side, as it will bring in the component of body image and left-right orientation. One point each (three points).
- **Obeying a written command**: Write in large letters 'close your eyes' (one point).
- **Repetition:** Ask the patient to say 'no ifs, ands or buts'.
- **Writing:** Ask the patient to write a sentence with a subject and object which makes sense. No marks are deleted for spelling errors (one point).
- **Drawing:** Ask the patient to draw a circle, square and a triangle (one point).

The maximum score is 30 points. Less than 24 means that there is a cognitive deficit.

INDEX